Dr. Henry plath

Ancient Natural Remed[ies]

with Modern Medicine

Combining Ancient Remedies Revived with Modern Medical Practices

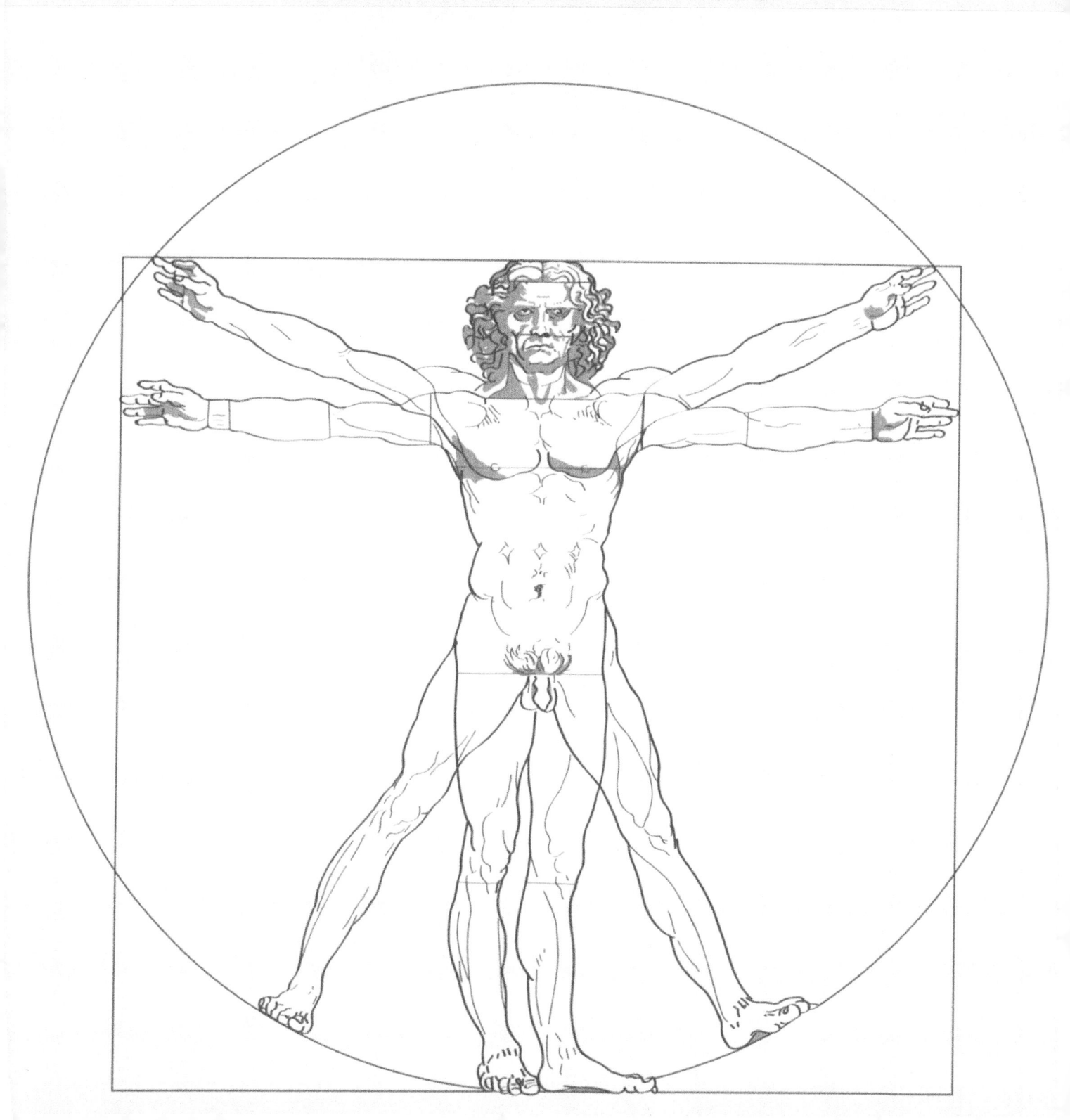

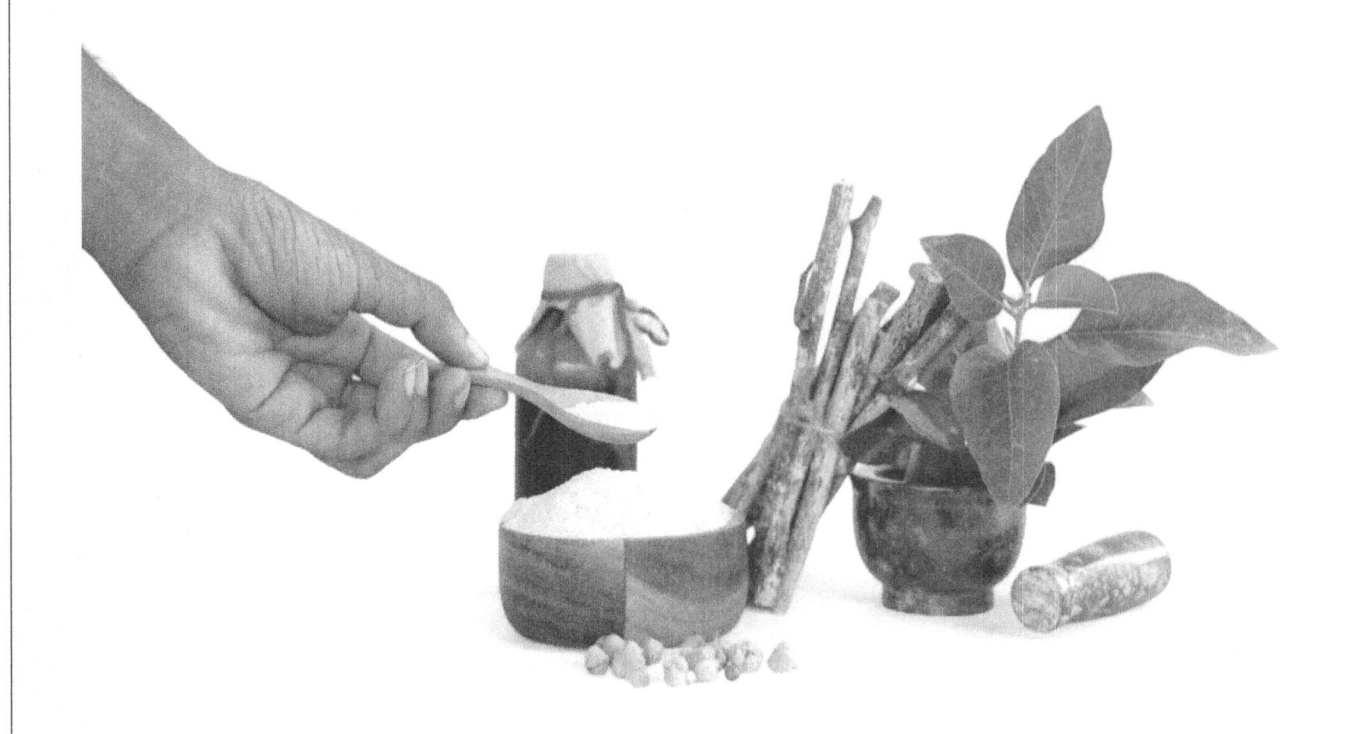

Biographical outline

Henry Plath, born in 1967 in Louisiana, is an award-winning physician, chef, and respected phytotherapy scholar, celebrated for his pioneering work linking the fields of medicine and culinary arts. A medical graduate with a specialization in nutrition, Plath has dedicated his career to exploring the therapeutic potential of food and natural remedies, particularly in the treatment and prevention of inflammatory diseases. His work integrates the principles of phytotherapy—a discipline focused on using plants and natural extracts to prevent and treat illness—demonstrating how nutrition can act as a powerful tool for health.

Plath conducted significant research at one of Louisiana's leading centers for native and medicinal plant studies, enhancing his expertise and understanding of how natural compounds can impact human health. His successful publications reflect his commitment to making nutritional science accessible through recipes and dietary plans that combine flavor with well-being. With numerous accolades for his innovative approach, Plath has become a leading figure in healthy cooking, inspiring a global audience to embrace a holistic approach to health and wellness.

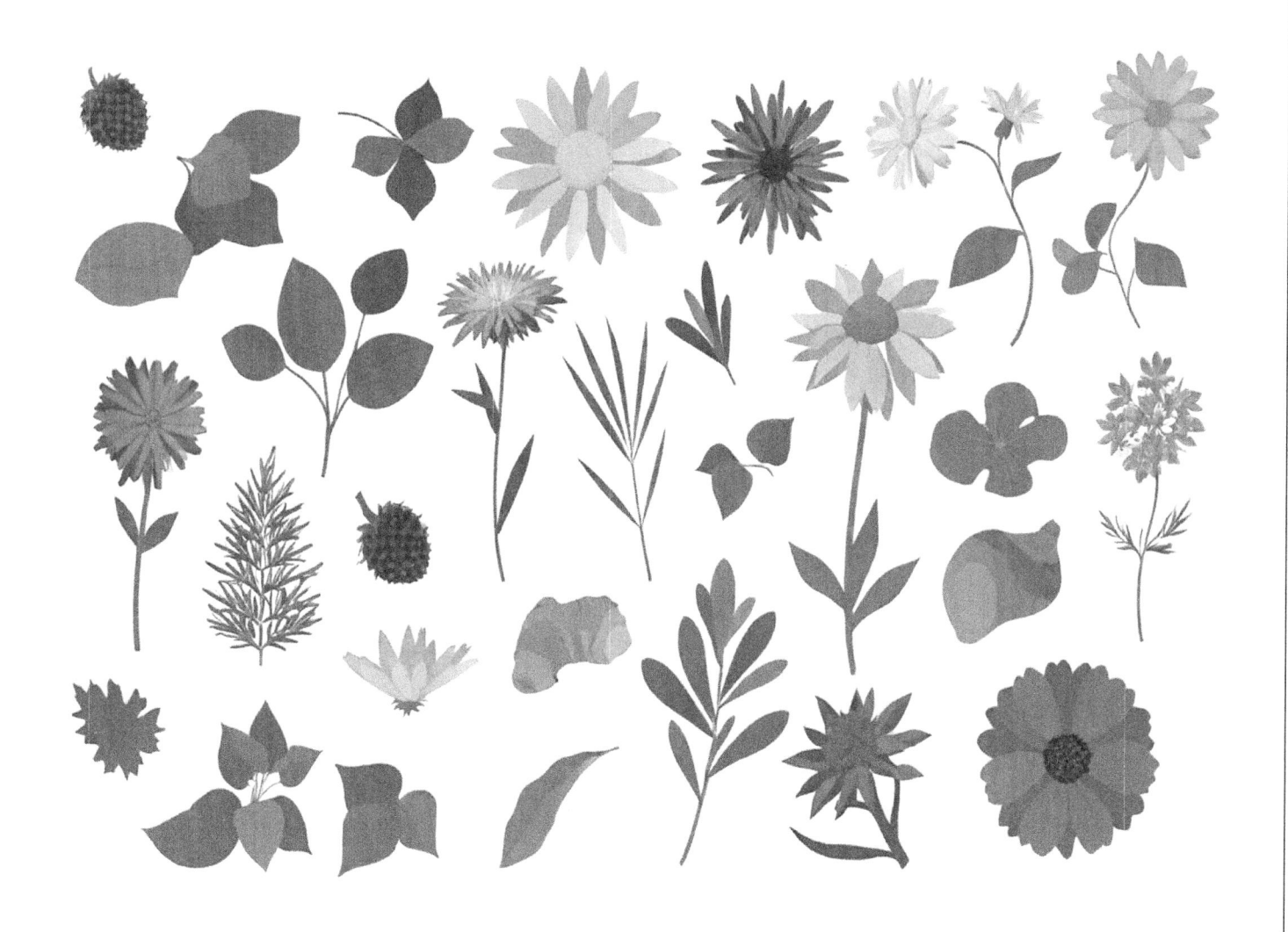

Disclaimer

This book, *Ancient Natural Remedies Improved with Modern Medicine*, is intended solely for informational and educational purposes. The content within is not meant to replace professional medical advice, diagnosis, or treatment. Readers are strongly encouraged to consult their doctor, nutritionist, or healthcare provider before making significant changes to their diet, lifestyle, or healthcare routines, particularly if they have pre-existing medical conditions, food allergies, intolerances, or are taking prescribed medications.

The remedies, recipes, and advice presented in this book are designed to explore the potential of natural and ancient healing practices alongside modern medicine. However, individual results may vary. The effectiveness of any remedy or dietary change depends on personal health factors, and we cannot guarantee specific outcomes related to improved health, reduced inflammation, or any other claims discussed. Readers are urged to carefully observe how their body responds to new practices or remedies and to discontinue use and seek professional medical advice if they experience any adverse reactions or concerns. The authors and publishers disclaim any liability for damages, injuries, or health complications arising from the application of information or recipes provided in this book.

This disclaimer serves to remind readers that their health and well-being require a personalized approach and that all remedies, supplements, or dietary changes should be undertaken responsibly and under the guidance of qualified healthcare professionals.

Index

Chapter 1 13

  The Legacy of Traditional Medicine 13

    Origins of Natural Remedies: Medicinal Plants, Essential Oils, and Holistic Therapies Used Across Various Cultures (e.g., Chinese, Ayurvedic, and Greek Medicine) 14

    What Makes These Remedies Effective: Natural Active Compounds, Their Effects on the Body, and Common Applications 15

    Limitations and Challenges: Lack of Standardization and Difficulty in Establishing Scientific Efficacy 16

  The Contribution of Modern Medicine 18

    Research and Development Methods: How Modern Medicine Analyzes and Isolates the Active Ingredients in Natural Remedies 18

    Modern Pharmacology: Exploring How Medications Are Based on Natural Compounds 20

Chapter 3 25

  Potent Medicinal Herbs and Plants 25

    Examples of Traditional Plants (Turmeric, Echinacea, Ginseng) and Their Natural Benefits 25

  Enhancing Health with Traditional Plants 27

    25 beneficial recipes for general health 27

Chapter 4 37

  Integrative Approaches to Well-being 37

    Combating Inflammation and Pain: The Use of Natural Remedies Like Devil's Claw and Modern Techniques to Enhance Relief 37

    Understanding Devil's Claw and Its Benefits 37

    Other Natural Remedies for Inflammation and Pain 37

    Modern Techniques to Enhance the Effectiveness of Natural Remedies 38

    Integrating Natural Remedies with Conventional Treatments 39

    Practical Considerations and Safety 39

    Dosage and Modern Variants: Utilizing Advanced Extraction Methods and Optimized Dosing 39

    Optimized Extraction Methods for Consistency and Potency 40

    Optimized Dosage for Maximum Effectiveness 40

    Customized Formulations and Delivery Methods 41

    The Role of Modern Research in Dosing Precision 42

    Safety and Precision: Ensuring Effective Natural Remedies 42

    Mental Health and Stress: Ancient Remedies for Calm and Sleep (Like Chamomile and Lavender) with the Support of Modern Techniques Like Biofeedback and Mindfulness 42

Ancient Remedies for Calm and Sleep 43

Modern Techniques to Enhance Mental Health and Manage Stress 43

Integrating Ancient Remedies and Modern Techniques for Comprehensive Stress Relief 44

Practical Tips for Using Ancient Remedies and Techniques Together 44

Digestion and Immunity: Traditional Uses of Natural Probiotics, Supported and Enhanced by Modern Science 45

Traditional Uses of Natural Probiotics 45

The Science Behind Probiotics and Their Role in Digestive and Immune Health 46

Modern Advancements in Probiotic Supplementation 47

Integrating Traditional and Modern Probiotics for Enhanced Health Benefits _____ 47

25 Natural recipes for pain and inflammation_____ 48

25 recipes for mental health and relaxation_____ 55

Chapter 5_____ 62

Natural Remedies and Skin Care_____ 62

For Skin Care: Traditional Treatments with Aloe Vera, Tea Tree, Coconut Oil, and Other Natural Remedies   62

Aloe Vera: The Healing Plant 62

Tea Tree Oil: Nature's Antimicrobial Powerhouse 62

Coconut Oil: The Deep Moisturizer 63

Other Natural Skin Remedies 63

How to Create a Simple Natural Skincare Routine 64

Modern Dermatology and Enhancements: How Modern Medicine Has Refined the Use of These Remedies for Specific Skin Issues like Acne, Wrinkles, and Irritations_____ 64

Aloe Vera for Acne and Skin Irritations 64

Tea Tree Oil for Acne and Oily Skin 65

Coconut Oil for Wrinkles and Dry Skin 65

Other Natural Ingredients Enhanced by Modern Dermatology 66

Combining Traditional Remedies with Advanced Dermatological Ingredients 66

Combined Skincare Routine: Practical Tips for Integrating Traditional Remedies and Modern Products_____67

Morning Routine 67

Evening Routine 68

General Tips for Combining Traditional and Modern Skincare 69

23 skin care recipes_____ 70

Chapter 6_____ 77

Natural Remedies and Cardiovascular Health_____ 77

Garlic: Nature's Heart Protector 77

Fish Oil: Rich in Heart-Healthy Omega-3 Fatty Acids 77

- Green Tea: A Powerful Antioxidant for Cardiovascular Support ... 78
- Integrating Garlic, Fish Oil, and Green Tea for Optimal Heart Health ... 79
  - Modern Research on Cardiovascular Benefits: Studies Supporting the Effectiveness of These Remedies ... 79
  - Garlic: Studies on Blood Pressure, Cholesterol, and Heart Health ... 79
  - Fish Oil: Omega-3 Fatty Acids and Cardiovascular Protection ... 80
  - Green Tea: Antioxidant-Rich Catechins and Heart Disease Prevention ... 80
  - Combined Effects and Synergistic Benefits ... 81
- Integrated Strategies for Heart Health: Combining Natural Remedies with Lifestyle Management and Medications, When Necessary ... 81
  - Natural Remedies for Heart Health ... 81
  - Lifestyle Adjustments for Optimal Heart Health ... 82
  - When Medications are Necessary ... 82
  - Building a Personalized Heart Health Plan ... 83
  - Heart-Healthy Recipes: Teas, Juices, and Dishes with Traditional Ingredients Like Garlic, Green Tea, and Fish Oil ... 84

25 recipes for the well-being of the heart ... 84

- Chapter 7 ... 91
- Energy Management and General Welfare ... 91
  - Remedies for Energy and Wellness: Ginseng, Ashwagandha, and Other Adaptogenic Herbs ... 91
  - Ginseng: The Vitality Herb ... 91
  - Ashwagandha: The Stress-Relieving Adaptogen ... 91
  - Rhodiola Rosea: The Endurance Enhancer ... 92
  - Holy Basil: The Calming Herb ... 92
  - Maca Root: The Energizing Root ... 93
  - Eleuthero: The Energy-Boosting Herb ... 93
  - Combining Adaptogens for Optimal Energy and Wellness ... 93
  - Precautions and Tips ... 94
  - Mechanisms of Action: Understanding How Adaptogens Work ... 94
  - Improved Safety and Quality Control in Adaptogenic Supplements ... 95
  - Clinical Studies Supporting the Safety of Adaptogens ... 95
  - Integrating Adaptogens Safely into Modern Health Practices ... 96
- Practical Tips for Integration: How to Choose the Best Products and Combine Them with Modern Lifestyle Strategies ... 97
  - Combining Adaptogens with Modern Lifestyle Practices ... 97
  - Personalizing Your Adaptogen Routine ... 98
  - Avoiding Potential Pitfalls and Optimizing Safety ... 99
  - Energizing and Revitalizing Recipes: Adaptogenic Beverages, Smoothies, and Snacks to Boost Energy and Overall Well-Being ... 100

25 recipes for mental well-being ... 100

Chapter 8 — 107

Myths and Truths about Natural Remedies — 107

Remedies That Really Work — 107
Remedies That Lack Strong Scientific Evidence — 108
Remedies That Show Potential But Need More Research — 110

Common Misconceptions: How to Avoid Traps and Myths About Natural Remedies — 111

"Natural" Means Safe — 111
More Is Better — 111
Natural Remedies Work Instantly — 112
All Health Claims Are Created Equal — 112
Traditional Use Equals Scientific Validation — 113
If It's a Popular Trend, It Must Work — 113
"All-Natural" Means It's Free of Harmful Ingredients — 113
One Remedy Works for Everyone — 114
Natural Remedies Don't Interact with Medications — 114
Natural Remedies Are a Substitute for Medical Treatment — 115

Verifying Sources and Products: Tips for Identifying Safe and Reliable Products — 115

Look for Third-Party Testing and Certifications — 115
Choose Products from Transparent, Reputable Brands — 116
Review the Ingredients and Avoid Unnecessary Additives — 116
Research the Manufacturer's Reputation and Track Record — 117
Understand the Dosage and Potency of Ingredients — 117
Verify Product Claims with Scientific Evidence — 118
Be Wary of Products That Are "Too Good to Be True" — 118
Consult a Healthcare Professional When in Doubt — 119
Buy from Trusted Sources and Retailers — 119
Track Your Experience and Results — 120

Chapter 9 — 121

Guidelines for Safe Use — 121

Understand Potential Interactions — 121
Consult Your Healthcare Provider — 121
Start Low and Go Slow — 122
Avoid "Stacking" Remedies with Similar Effects — 122
Time Dosing Carefully — 122
Stick to Recommended Dosages — 123
Monitor for Side Effects and Adjust as Needed — 123
Choose Reputable Sources and High-Quality Products — 123
Consider Cycling or "Taking Breaks" — 124
Know When to Avoid Combining Remedies and Medications — 124

- Use Natural Remedies to Complement, Not Replace, Medications 124
- Seek Professional Guidance with Complex Health Conditions 125

Warnings and Contraindications: Identifying Dangerous Interactions and Recognizing When to Consult a Doctor 125

- Be Aware of Herb-Drug Interactions 125
- Recognize Conditions that May Be Worsened by Natural Remedies 126
- Be Cautious with Remedies That Affect Blood Clotting 127
- Watch for Central Nervous System Interactions 127
- Why It Matters: 127
- Know When Natural Remedies May Impact Hormone Levels 128
- Avoid Supplements with Undefined Ingredients or "Proprietary Blends" 128
- Why It Matters: 128
- Recognize When Symptoms Worsen and Seek Help Immediately 128
- Why It Matters: 128
- Be Cautious with "Detox" or "Cleansing" Supplements 129
- Know When to Consult a Healthcare Provider 129
- Be Open with Your Healthcare Team 129
- Start with Clear Health Goals 130
- Build a Daily Routine for Consistency 131
- Start with One Remedy at a Time 131
- Use Reliable Sources for Research 131
- Keep an Open Dialogue with Your Healthcare Provider 132
- Be Mindful of Possible Side Effects and Interactions 132
- Plan Around Your Medications 132
- Understand When It's Best to Avoid Certain Remedies 133
- Common Questions About Combining Natural Remedies and Medications 133
- Use Technology to Support Your Routine 134
- Be Patient and Flexible with Your Health Journey 134
- Trust Your Body and Seek Guidance When Needed 134

Introduction:

A Journey Through the Evolution of Medicine

Welcome to **"Ancient Natural Remedies Improved with Modern Medicine"**, a comprehensive guide that stands as a quintessential **Ancient Remedies Revived book**, merging traditional wisdom with contemporary science to promote a healthier life.

The story of medicine is a fascinating journey, deeply intertwined with the wisdom of natural remedies. For millennia, these remedies have been the cornerstone of healing practices worldwide, shaping traditional medicine systems unique to each culture. By delving into this rich history, we uncover how ancient remedies—crafted long before modern technology—laid the groundwork for the advanced medical practices we rely on today.

Imagine ancient Egypt, where healers harnessed the antibacterial power of garlic and honey to treat wounds and infections. The **Ebers Papyrus**, a treasure trove of herbal remedies dating back thousands of years, reveals a remarkable sophistication in health and healing that continues to inspire modern herbal medicine.

Travel to China, where over 2,500 years ago, the principles of Traditional Chinese Medicine emerged, introducing practices like acupuncture and herbal therapy. Ingredients such as ginseng, known for enhancing vitality, and liquorice root, prized for immune support, are enduring legacies of this ancient knowledge, still embraced globally.

In India, the holistic world of **Ayurveda** seamlessly blends nutrition, meditation, and medicinal plants. The golden hues of turmeric, revered for its anti-inflammatory properties, and the calming power of ashwagandha, used to balance stress, highlight the ingenuity of a system that views wellness as a harmony of body, mind, and spirit.

Embarking on this journey through the evolution of medicine offers more than just historical insight—it reconnects us with nature's power to heal and inspires us to integrate ancient wisdom into our modern lives. This **Ancient Remedies Revived book** is your gateway to understanding the timeless connection between humanity and the healing gifts of the earth.

Overview of the Evolution of Medicine: A Brief History of Natural Remedies and Their Use Across Cultures

The evolution of medicine is deeply intertwined with the development and use of natural remedies. For thousands of years, natural substances derived from plants, minerals, and animal products have been used in healing practices around the world. Each culture, drawing on local resources and traditional knowledge passed down through generations, developed unique systems of natural medicine that laid the foundation for modern medical science. By exploring this history, we can gain insight into how ancient remedies—despite being crafted without the benefit of today's technologies—have influenced and informed modern approaches to health and wellness.

In ancient Egypt, healers employed herbs like garlic and honey for their antibacterial and antiseptic properties. Texts such as the Ebers Papyrus, one of the oldest known medical manuscripts, document hundreds of herbal remedies and natural therapies, highlighting an advanced understanding of disease prevention and treatment in early Egyptian society.

Traditional Chinese medicine (TCM), which has roots stretching back over 2,500 years, introduced practices such as acupuncture, herbal medicine, and the concept of balancing "Qi" or life energy. Herbs like ginseng and licorice root were used to promote vitality and strengthen the immune system—remedies that remain popular today due to centuries of use and study.

In India, Ayurveda, a holistic system of medicine, emphasized balance in body, mind, and spirit. This ancient practice utilized a variety of plants, such as turmeric and ashwagandha, to treat a wide range of health issues. Ayurveda combined herbal treatments with dietary guidelines and lifestyle practices, creating an integrated approach to health that remains relevant today.

Similarly, in ancient Greece, Hippocrates—known as the father of modern medicine—promoted the use of natural substances like willow bark (the precursor to modern aspirin) to relieve pain and inflammation. His teachings laid the groundwork for a system of medicine that values natural, whole-body treatments. While these ancient systems were distinct in their practices and philosophies, they shared a common view: that true health requires treating both the body and the mind. Over centuries, as modern medicine began to develop with a focus on empirical evidence and scientific discovery, natural remedies continued to play a significant role. Today, advances in research allow us to isolate the active compounds within traditional remedies, enhancing their efficacy and ensuring their safety.

This overview of the evolution of medicine demonstrates that, although science has made incredible progress, the roots of medicine remain closely tied to natural healing practices. Today, the trend towards integrative medicine acknowledges the value of combining ancient traditions with modern scientific advancements, offering a balanced approach to achieving optimal health.

Goal of the Book: To Explain How Modern Medicine Can Enhance and Support the Effectiveness of Traditional Natural Remedies

The primary goal of this book is to offer a comprehensive guide on how modern medicine can not only coexist with traditional natural remedies but can also amplify their effectiveness, making them safer, more precise, and more accessible. In recent decades, science has made remarkable advances in understanding the active components that make many plants, herbs, and other natural substances beneficial for health. Through these discoveries, we are now able to improve their therapeutic potential with innovations in standardization, optimal dosing, and the creation of more effective formulations.

This book will explore how scientific research has identified and isolated the active ingredients in traditional remedies, enhancing their action while reducing potential side effects. We'll discuss how modern technologies, such as cold extraction, controlled dosing techniques, and pharmacological engineering, are transforming natural medicine to offer targeted and sustainable benefits for a wide range of conditions, from general wellness to the management of chronic issues.

Furthermore, the book will examine how combining natural remedies with medical treatments can provide an integrated and powerful solution, capable of addressing health concerns in a holistic manner. Integrative approaches allow us to benefit from the complementary strengths of both methodologies: natural remedies provide gentle, gradual support, while modern medicine offers precision and rapid action. This combination is particularly effective in areas such as immune support, stress management, cardiovascular health, and mental wellness.

The ultimate aim is to guide readers toward a responsible and informed use of both natural and medical treatments, inspiring a health approach that does not separate traditional practices from scientific advancements, but instead unites them in a synergy capable of improving quality of life.

The Importance of Integration: How and Why to Combine the Best of Both Worlds for Enhanced Health and Well-being

In recent years, there has been a growing recognition of the importance of integrating traditional natural remedies with modern medicine to achieve better health outcomes and improve overall well-being. This approach, often referred to as integrative or complementary medicine, brings together the time-tested benefits of natural remedies with the precision, efficiency, and scientific rigor of modern medical practices. By combining these two worlds, we can create a more balanced, holistic approach to health that addresses the needs of the whole person—body, mind, and spirit.

One of the key reasons to integrate natural remedies with modern medicine is that each system has its strengths and limitations. Traditional remedies, which often use plants, herbs, and other natural substances, provide gentle and sustained support for the body's natural healing processes. They are typically less invasive and have fewer side effects compared to many conventional treatments. However, natural remedies can sometimes lack the potency or specificity needed to address severe or acute health issues quickly. This is where modern medicine excels, with its targeted therapies, scientifically tested medications, and advanced diagnostic tools.

By integrating natural remedies with modern medical treatments, we are able to create a more personalized and effective approach to health. For example, someone managing chronic pain might benefit from the anti-inflammatory properties of natural herbs like turmeric, combined with the precision of pharmaceutical pain relievers for immediate relief when needed. Similarly, stress and anxiety can be managed through both calming herbal teas and scientifically backed practices like mindfulness, biofeedback, or even medication if necessary. This approach not only allows for more effective treatment but also promotes long-term wellness by supporting both immediate needs and underlying health.

Another significant advantage of this integrative approach is that it empowers individuals to take a proactive role in their own health. By incorporating natural remedies, people can make lifestyle adjustments and introduce daily habits that enhance their well-being, rather than relying solely on medical interventions. This sense of control and self-care can lead to better health outcomes, as individuals are more engaged and committed to their health journey.

Overall, the integration of natural remedies with modern medicine allows us to leverage the best of both worlds. It creates a comprehensive approach to health that is not only effective in addressing symptoms but also sustainable in promoting long-term well-being. In a world where health needs are complex and varied, this balanced approach provides a way to address individual needs while honoring both traditional wisdom and modern advancements.

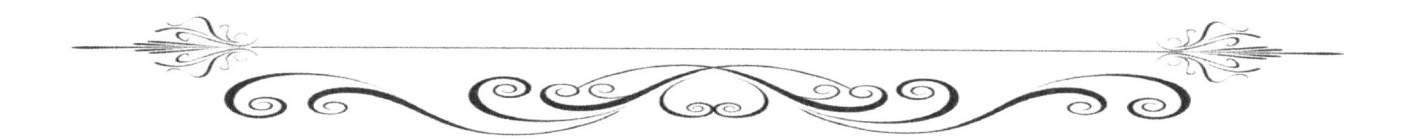

Chapter 1

The Legacy of Traditional Medicine

Origins of Natural Remedies: Medicinal Plants, Essential Oils, and Holistic Therapies Used Across Various Cultures (e.g., Chinese, Ayurvedic, and Greek Medicine)

The origins of natural remedies are deeply rooted in the history of human civilization, with medicinal plants, essential oils, and holistic therapies forming the foundation of healthcare practices in diverse cultures around the world. These early healing systems developed out of necessity, curiosity, and the human desire to alleviate suffering, resulting in rich traditions that continue to influence natural medicine today. Each culture, with its unique environment, resources, and worldview, developed distinct approaches to natural healing that have contributed to the collective wisdom we rely on in integrative medicine.

In **Traditional Chinese Medicine (TCM)**, the use of natural remedies can be traced back over 2,500 years. Chinese healers developed a highly sophisticated system of medicine based on the concept of balancing the body's vital energy, or *Qi*, which flows through pathways known as meridians. By using herbs, acupuncture, and dietary therapies, TCM aims to restore harmony within the body, which is believed to be the key to health. Medicinal plants like **ginseng**, known for boosting energy, **gingko biloba**, which supports brain health, and **licorice root**, used to harmonize other herbal ingredients, have become staples in TCM. This traditional system also employs essential oils like **eucalyptus** and **tea tree** for respiratory health and immune support.

In **Ayurvedic medicine**, which originated in India over 3,000 years ago, health is viewed as a delicate balance between the body, mind, and spirit. Ayurveda emphasizes natural remedies that are tailored to each individual's unique constitution, or *dosha*, with the goal of creating harmony between the internal and external environments. Medicinal plants like **turmeric**, with its powerful anti-inflammatory properties, **ashwagandha**, which aids in stress management, and **holy basil** (tulsi), known for its immune-boosting effects, are fundamental to Ayurvedic practices. Essential oils such as **sandalwood** for mental clarity and **jasmine** for mood enhancement are also widely used in Ayurvedic healing, often in combination with massage and other body therapies to promote balance and well-being.

In **Ancient Greek medicine**, natural remedies were highly valued and carefully studied by influential figures such as Hippocrates, often referred to as the "Father of Medicine." Greek healers believed in the body's ability to heal itself with the help of nature, and they employed medicinal plants like **willow bark**, the precursor to aspirin, for pain relief, and **garlic**, valued for its antibacterial and cardiovascular benefits. Greek medicine also placed a strong emphasis on the role of diet and lifestyle in health, often using herbal infusions and essential oils like

lavender for relaxation and **rosemary** for memory and cognitive support. This focus on preventative care, combined with the use of natural substances, laid the groundwork for Western herbalism and holistic practices.

Each of these healing traditions—Chinese, Ayurvedic, and Greek—developed a comprehensive approach to health that focused not only on treating symptoms but also on maintaining balance, preventing illness, and promoting long-term well-being. By drawing on the wisdom of nature, they have provided powerful, effective remedies that continue to support health worldwide. Today, these traditional approaches remain highly regarded, and their influence can be seen in modern integrative medicine, where the principles of balance, natural healing, and prevention continue to guide us in caring for both body and mind.

Origins of Natural Remedies: Medicinal Plants, Essential Oils, and Holistic Therapies Used Across Various Cultures (e.g., Chinese, Ayurvedic, and Greek Medicine)

The origins of natural remedies are deeply rooted in the history of human civilization, with medicinal plants, essential oils, and holistic therapies forming the foundation of healthcare practices in diverse cultures around the world. These early healing systems developed out of necessity, curiosity, and the human desire to alleviate suffering, resulting in rich traditions that continue to influence natural medicine today. Each culture, with its unique environment, resources, and worldview, developed distinct approaches to natural healing that have contributed to the collective wisdom we rely on in integrative medicine.

In **Traditional Chinese Medicine (TCM)**, the use of natural remedies can be traced back over 2,500 years. Chinese healers developed a highly sophisticated system of medicine based on the concept of balancing the body's vital energy, or *Qi*, which flows through pathways known as meridians. By using herbs, acupuncture, and dietary therapies, TCM aims to restore harmony within the body, which is believed to be the key to health. Medicinal plants like **ginseng**, known for boosting energy, **gingko biloba**, which supports brain health, and **licorice root**, used to harmonize other herbal ingredients, have become staples in TCM. This traditional system also employs essential oils like **eucalyptus** and **tea tree** for respiratory health and immune support.

In **Ayurvedic medicine**, which originated in India over 3,000 years ago, health is viewed as a delicate balance between the body, mind, and spirit. Ayurveda emphasizes natural remedies that are tailored to each individual's unique constitution, or *dosha*, with the goal of creating harmony between the internal and external environments. Medicinal plants like **turmeric**, with its powerful anti-inflammatory properties, **ashwagandha**, which aids in stress management, and **holy basil** (tulsi), known for its immune-boosting effects, are fundamental to Ayurvedic practices. Essential oils such as **sandalwood** for mental clarity and **jasmine** for mood enhancement are also widely used in Ayurvedic healing, often in combination with massage and other body therapies to promote balance and well-being.

In **Ancient Greek medicine**, natural remedies were highly valued and carefully studied by influential figures such as Hippocrates, often referred to as the "Father of Medicine." Greek healers believed in the body's ability to heal itself with the help of nature, and they employed medicinal plants like **willow bark**, the precursor to aspirin, for pain relief, and **garlic**, valued for its antibacterial and cardiovascular benefits. Greek medicine also placed a strong emphasis on the role of diet and lifestyle in health, often using herbal infusions and essential oils like **lavender** for relaxation and **rosemary** for memory and cognitive support. This focus on preventative care, combined with the use of natural substances, laid the groundwork for Western herbalism and holistic practices.

Each of these healing traditions—Chinese, Ayurvedic, and Greek—developed a comprehensive approach to health that focused not only on treating symptoms but also on maintaining balance, preventing illness, and promoting long-term well-being. By drawing on the wisdom of nature, they have provided powerful, effective remedies that continue to support health worldwide. Today, these traditional approaches remain highly regarded, and their influence can be seen in modern integrative medicine, where the principles of balance, natural healing, and prevention continue to guide us in caring for both body and mind.

What Makes These Remedies Effective: Natural Active Compounds, Their Effects on the Body, and Common   Applications

The effectiveness of natural remedies lies in their unique active compounds, which interact with the body in ways that support healing and well-being. Unlike synthetic drugs, which often target specific symptoms or functions, natural remedies tend to work holistically, offering a range of benefits that can positively impact multiple systems within the body. These remedies have been used and refined over centuries, and their active ingredients—phytochemicals, essential oils, antioxidants, and minerals—contribute to their powerful effects on the body.

1. Natural Active Compounds

Medicinal plants and other natural substances are effective largely due to their active compounds, which are naturally occurring chemicals that support health. For instance, the **curcuminoids** in turmeric provide anti-inflammatory and antioxidant effects, helping to reduce inflammation in the body. **Alkaloids** in plants like echinacea stimulate the immune system, increasing the body's ability to ward off infections. **Polyphenols** and **flavonoids** found in green tea and other plants have strong antioxidant properties, protecting cells from damage caused by free radicals. These natural compounds often work synergistically, meaning they enhance each other's effectiveness when combined, leading to a more powerful impact on health.

2. Effects on the Body

The active ingredients in natural remedies interact with the body's systems in various ways, often helping to restore balance and promote natural healing. For example, certain compounds found in plants like valerian and chamomile have a calming effect on the central nervous system, making them effective in managing stress and promoting relaxation. Others, like the **glycyrrhizin** in licorice root, have anti-inflammatory and soothing effects on the digestive tract, making it beneficial for gastrointestinal health. These natural compounds often provide benefits that are both immediate and long-lasting, supporting overall wellness rather than just symptom relief.

Furthermore, natural remedies can stimulate the body's self-healing processes. **Adaptogens** like ashwagandha and ginseng, for instance, help the body respond better to stress by regulating the adrenal glands and balancing hormone levels, which supports resilience and energy over time. Essential oils such as **peppermint** and **lavender** also have a range of applications, from easing headaches and improving mental clarity to promoting sleep and reducing anxiety. By working in harmony with the body, these remedies promote a state of equilibrium, which is essential for long-term health.

3. Common Applications

Natural remedies are widely used for a variety of common health concerns, including pain relief, immune support, mental well-being, and digestive health. Herbal teas, tinctures, and essential oils are common forms in which these remedies are used, as they offer easy and accessible ways to benefit from the plants' active compounds. For instance, ginger is widely used for nausea and digestive support, while garlic is known for its cardiovascular and immune-boosting properties. These remedies are often versatile; turmeric, for example, is used not only for its anti-inflammatory effects but also for its support in joint health and liver function.

Due to their broad range of effects, natural remedies are also commonly used as preventive tools to maintain wellness and support the body's resilience. They can be easily integrated into daily routines, such as drinking herbal teas for relaxation or incorporating immune-boosting spices like garlic and ginger into meals. For chronic issues, natural remedies can be combined with conventional treatments, often enhancing their effectiveness or reducing the side effects of pharmaceuticals.

In summary, natural remedies are effective because they contain active compounds that interact beneficially with the body's systems, promote balance, and support holistic health. Their versatility, safety, and broad application make them valuable tools in both preventive care and the treatment of various ailments. These natural substances have stood the test of time due to their ability to promote healing in a way that complements the body's innate processes, making them an essential component of integrative health practices today.

Limitations and Challenges: Lack of Standardization and Difficulty in Establishing Scientific Efficacy

Despite their long history of use and the widespread appeal of natural remedies, there are significant limitations and challenges that come with their application in modern healthcare. Two of the primary challenges include the lack of standardization and the difficulty of establishing scientific efficacy. Understanding these issues is essential for anyone interested in integrating natural remedies into a holistic healthcare approach, as they can impact both the reliability and safety of these treatments.

1. Lack of Standardization

One of the most significant limitations of natural remedies is the lack of standardization. Unlike pharmaceuticals, which are manufactured under strict quality controls to ensure consistent potency and dosage, natural remedies can vary widely in strength and composition depending on factors such as the plant species, growing conditions, and methods of harvesting and processing. For example, the active compounds in a plant may differ in concentration based on the soil quality, climate, and season when it was harvested. Additionally, different manufacturers may use various extraction methods or add other ingredients that can alter the potency and effectiveness of the remedy.

This lack of standardization poses a challenge for both healthcare providers and patients. Without a consistent measure of strength and dosage, it is difficult to determine the correct amount to use, which can impact the effectiveness of the remedy and potentially lead to unwanted side effects. For example, a high concentration of active compounds may cause adverse reactions, while a low concentration may not provide the desired therapeutic effect. In contrast, standardized extracts—where the amount of active compound is controlled and consistent across batches—are more reliable but are not always available or affordable for all types of natural remedies.

2. Difficulty in Establishing Scientific Efficacy

Another major challenge with natural remedies is the difficulty in establishing scientific efficacy. While traditional knowledge and anecdotal evidence suggest that many natural remedies can be beneficial, rigorous scientific studies are often lacking or inconclusive. Scientific studies require large, controlled trials to reliably determine if a remedy is effective, but these trials can be costly and time-consuming. Additionally, natural substances are complex mixtures of various compounds, making it difficult to isolate the specific ingredient responsible for a particular therapeutic effect.

In modern medicine, the gold standard for demonstrating efficacy is the randomized controlled trial (RCT), which minimizes bias and provides clear data on a treatment's effectiveness. However, conducting RCTs for natural remedies presents several challenges. For instance, many plants and herbs contain multiple active compounds that work together, making it hard to determine which compound is responsible for the effects or how different compounds may work synergistically. Furthermore, the placebo effect can be particularly strong in natural medicine, as users often believe strongly in the effectiveness of natural treatments, which can skew results.

Due to these challenges, many natural remedies have not been subjected to the same level of scientific scrutiny as conventional medications. This lack of evidence can make it difficult for healthcare providers to confidently recommend natural remedies to patients, and it may lead to skepticism among patients who prioritize evidence-based treatments. While some natural remedies have gained support from smaller studies, the evidence is often not strong enough to meet the standards required for mainstream medical approval.

3. Quality Control and Regulatory Challenges

The lack of standardization and scientific efficacy is further complicated by regulatory challenges. In many countries, natural remedies are regulated as dietary supplements rather than medications, which means they are not subject to the same rigorous testing and approval processes as pharmaceutical drugs. As a result, there can be a wide variation in product quality, with some products containing contaminants or incorrect labeling of the active ingredients. Without strict oversight, it is difficult to ensure that consumers are receiving safe and effective products, which can undermine the credibility of natural remedies as a whole.

4. Moving Toward Solutions

Addressing these limitations requires a multi-faceted approach. Efforts are underway in some parts of the world to improve the standardization and quality control of natural remedies, with organizations working to develop guidelines for the cultivation, harvesting, and processing of medicinal plants. Scientific research is also gradually expanding to include more rigorous studies on natural remedies, aiming to isolate active compounds, understand their mechanisms of action, and conduct larger trials to assess efficacy.

While there is still progress to be made, an increasing number of standardized herbal products and natural extracts are becoming available. For users of natural remedies, choosing products from reputable brands with quality certifications and transparency about ingredient sourcing can also help mitigate some of these challenges.

In summary, while natural remedies offer promising health benefits, limitations like lack of standardization and difficulty in establishing scientific efficacy remain substantial obstacles. Overcoming these challenges will require continued research, improved regulations, and an ongoing commitment to balancing traditional knowledge with scientific rigor to ensure the safe and effective integration of natural remedies in modern healthcare practices.

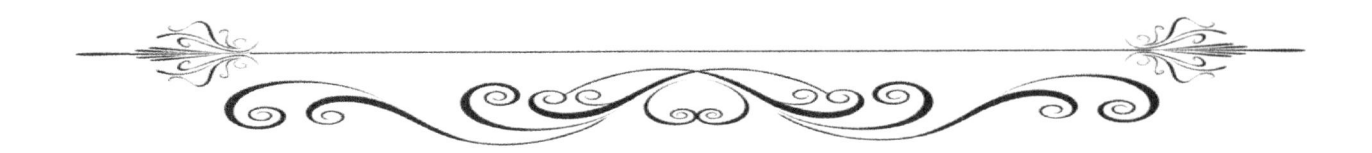

Chapter 2

The Contribution of Modern Medicine

Research and Development Methods: How Modern Medicine Analyzes and Isolates the Active Ingredients in Natural Remedies

Modern medicine has made great strides in harnessing the power of natural remedies by employing sophisticated research and development methods to analyze and isolate their active ingredients. By breaking down complex natural substances and studying their individual components, scientists are able to better understand the mechanisms behind their therapeutic effects, ensure consistent potency, and develop more targeted treatments. These advances in research and development have brought a level of precision to natural medicine that was not previously possible, helping to bridge the gap between traditional practices and scientifically-backed healthcare.

1. **Identifying Active Compounds**
   One of the primary goals in the study of natural remedies is identifying the specific active compounds responsible for their healing effects. Plants, herbs, and other natural sources contain a wide variety of bioactive compounds, such as alkaloids, flavonoids, polyphenols, terpenes, and essential oils. These compounds often work together synergistically, contributing to the overall efficacy of the remedy. Using analytical techniques like **mass spectrometry**, **high-performance liquid chromatography (HPLC)**, and **gas chromatography**, researchers can isolate and quantify these compounds. By identifying the most potent and beneficial compounds, scientists can focus their efforts on understanding how these individual molecules interact with the body.

2. **Extracting and Purifying Active Ingredients**
   Once the key active compounds are identified, the next step is to extract and purify them to create a concentrated form of the remedy that maximizes its effectiveness. Various extraction techniques are used depending on the nature of the compound, including **solvent extraction**, **cold pressing**, **steam distillation**, and **supercritical CO2 extraction**. Supercritical CO2 extraction, for instance, is a highly effective method for obtaining pure extracts without leaving harmful residues, making it ideal for delicate compounds like essential oils and flavonoids. These techniques help ensure that the final product is potent, pure, and consistent in quality, allowing for more reliable and standardized natural remedies.

3. **Standardizing Dosages and Potency**
   Standardization is a crucial step in the development of natural remedies, as it ensures that each dose contains a consistent amount of active compounds. Unlike traditional methods, where the potency of natural substances could vary widely, modern medicine aims to provide

standardized extracts that deliver predictable and reproducible effects. Standardization involves adjusting the concentration of active ingredients in a product to meet a specific therapeutic threshold. For example, a standardized turmeric extract might contain a fixed percentage of curcuminoids, the active anti-inflammatory compounds, making it easier for healthcare providers to recommend precise dosages and for patients to experience consistent results.

4. **Studying Mechanisms of Action**
Understanding how a natural remedy works in the body, or its mechanism of action, is a critical part of modern research. Through
in vitro (test tube) and **in vivo** (animal or human) studies, scientists explore how active compounds interact with biological pathways. For example, research on the herb ginseng has revealed its effects on the adrenal glands and immune system, which helps explain its role as an adaptogen in managing stress. Similarly, compounds in garlic have been shown to support cardiovascular health by affecting blood pressure and cholesterol levels. These studies not only validate the traditional uses of natural remedies but also provide insights into their broader health benefits, which can lead to new therapeutic applications.

5. **Clinical Trials and Efficacy Testing**
To establish the safety and efficacy of natural remedies for human use, clinical trials are conducted. Clinical trials, typically divided into **Phase I, II, and III**, assess the effects of an extract or purified compound on human subjects in a controlled environment. In these trials, researchers look for positive effects on specific health conditions, monitor for any adverse reactions, and compare the results to those of placebo groups or conventional treatments. Clinical trials are essential for confirming the benefits of natural remedies and for obtaining regulatory approval, which allows them to be marketed as evidence-based therapies.

6. **Developing New Derivatives and Synthetic Analogues**
In some cases, once the active ingredients of a natural remedy have been isolated and studied, researchers may develop synthetic analogues or derivatives. Synthetic analogues are modified versions of the original compound that may offer enhanced potency, stability, or bioavailability. For example, aspirin was developed as a synthetic version of the salicin found in willow bark, providing a more reliable and easily dosed pain reliever. Similarly, researchers are exploring synthetic forms of compounds in traditional remedies like curcumin (from turmeric) to improve its absorption and make it more effective in treating inflammatory diseases. These derivatives can expand the therapeutic potential of natural remedies while offering the benefits of modern pharmaceutical formulations.

7. **Quality Control and Safety Testing**
A critical component of developing natural remedies is ensuring their safety for human consumption. Rigorous quality control testing is applied to raw materials and finished products to detect contaminants such as pesticides, heavy metals, and microbial impurities. Stability testing is also conducted to determine the shelf life of the product and ensure that its potency remains consistent over time. These quality control measures are essential for building trust in natural remedies as safe, effective options within modern healthcare.

8. **Integrating Data for Evidence-Based Recommendations**
The data gathered from these research and development processes is then compiled to provide healthcare professionals with evidence-based information on the use of natural

remedies. By creating detailed profiles of each remedy, including standardized dosages, known mechanisms of action, and clinical trial results, modern medicine offers a more scientific and precise approach to recommending natural treatments. This evidence-based approach enables practitioners to confidently integrate natural remedies into treatment plans, complementing conventional therapies with the benefits of traditional healing.

In conclusion, modern medicine's research and development methods have significantly advanced the field of natural remedies. By analyzing, isolating, and standardizing active ingredients, scientists are able to refine and optimize traditional treatments for use in today's healthcare system. This fusion of traditional wisdom and scientific rigor not only enhances the safety and efficacy of natural remedies but also ensures that they remain a valuable resource in promoting holistic health and well-being.

Modern Pharmacology: Exploring How Medications Are Based on Natural Compounds

Modern pharmacology, the science of drugs and their effects on the human body, has deep roots in the natural world. Many of the medications we rely on today were either directly derived from natural compounds or inspired by them. For centuries, healers and scientists have studied plants, minerals, and other natural resources to discover their healing properties. These discoveries have shaped the development of modern medicine, leading to the isolation and synthesis of powerful compounds that serve as the foundation for many pharmaceuticals in use today. By examining how medications are based on natural compounds, we gain insight into the intersection of traditional wisdom and scientific innovation, as well as the ongoing importance of nature in drug development.

1. **Natural Compounds as Drug Precursors**
   A significant portion of modern medications originated as compounds found in nature. Plants, fungi, marine organisms, and even microorganisms have provided valuable bioactive compounds that were later refined or synthesized to become mainstream drugs. One of the most well-known examples is **aspirin**, derived from salicin, a compound found in willow bark. For centuries, willow bark was used as a natural remedy for pain and fever, and in the 19th century, scientists identified and modified salicin to create acetylsalicylic acid, or aspirin, one of the most widely used medications in the world.

Another notable example is **morphine**, isolated from the opium poppy. For thousands of years, opium was used as a pain reliever, but the isolation of morphine allowed for a more controlled and potent analgesic that revolutionized pain management. The isolation of active ingredients from plants has allowed pharmacologists to create targeted therapies, taking advantage of nature's vast library of compounds.

2. **Discovery of Antibiotics from Natural Sources**
   One of the greatest medical breakthroughs of the 20th century, the discovery of antibiotics, also has natural origins. **Penicillin**, the first antibiotic, was discovered when Alexander Fleming observed that a mold, *Penicillium notatum*, inhibited the growth of bacteria. This discovery led to the development of penicillin-based antibiotics, which transformed medicine by providing effective treatments for bacterial infections. Since then, other

antibiotics derived from natural sources, such as **streptomycin** from soil bacteria, have been developed, showcasing nature's role in providing the raw materials for lifesaving drugs.

3. **Plants as a Source of Cancer Treatments**
Several groundbreaking cancer treatments have also been derived from natural sources. For instance, **taxol** (paclitaxel), a powerful chemotherapy agent, was originally extracted from the bark of the Pacific yew tree. Taxol has since become a critical drug in the treatment of various cancers, particularly breast and ovarian cancer. Similarly, **vincristine** and **vinblastine**, chemotherapy drugs used to treat leukemia and lymphoma, were discovered in the Madagascar periwinkle plant. These natural compounds inhibit the growth of cancer cells and have become cornerstones in oncology, highlighting how the search for effective cancer treatments often leads back to the natural world.

4. **Synthetic Analogues Inspired by Natural Compounds**
In many cases, scientists have created synthetic versions or analogues of natural compounds to improve their efficacy, stability, or safety. Synthetic analogues are chemically modified versions of naturally occurring compounds designed to retain the therapeutic benefits while overcoming limitations like poor absorption or toxicity. For example, many **opioid painkillers** are synthetic derivatives of morphine, developed to provide effective pain relief with modified effects. These analogues allow for more controlled effects and targeted action, demonstrating how natural compounds can serve as starting points for advanced pharmaceutical development.

5. **Natural Compounds in Cardiovascular Medicine**
Natural compounds have also had a profound impact on cardiovascular medicine. **Digitalis**, a compound derived from the foxglove plant, has been used for centuries to treat heart failure. Modern pharmacology isolated and refined digitalis into **digoxin**, a medication that helps strengthen heart contractions and regulate heartbeat in patients with heart conditions. Similarly, **statins**, cholesterol-lowering drugs, were inspired by compounds produced by fungi. Statins have become essential in the treatment of high cholesterol and heart disease, illustrating how naturally occurring molecules have paved the way for treatments in cardiology.

6. **Advances in Anti-Malarial Drugs from Nature**
Another area where natural compounds have made a lasting impact is in the treatment of malaria. **Quinine**, derived from the bark of the cinchona tree, was historically used to treat malaria, and it became the foundation for the development of synthetic antimalarial drugs. More recently, **artemisinin**, a compound isolated from the sweet wormwood plant, has become a cornerstone in malaria treatment. Artemisinin and its derivatives are highly effective against malaria parasites, and their discovery was a significant breakthrough in the fight against the disease.

7. **Marine and Microbial Sources of New Drugs**
The ocean and microbial world offer rich, largely untapped sources of new drugs. Marine organisms, such as sponges, corals, and algae, have yielded compounds with anti-inflammatory, antiviral, and anticancer properties. For instance, **cytarabine**, a chemotherapy drug used to treat leukemia, was derived from a compound found in sea sponges. Additionally, microbial sources, including soil bacteria, have led to the discovery of immunosuppressants like **cyclosporine**, which revolutionized organ transplantation by

preventing rejection. These discoveries underscore the vast potential of exploring diverse ecosystems for new medications.

8. **Challenges and Future Directions**

    While natural compounds have been instrumental in drug development, there are challenges associated with their use. Isolating and producing these compounds in sufficient quantities can be difficult, particularly when sourcing from endangered species or fragile ecosystems. Additionally, not all natural compounds can be easily synthesized, and some may have toxic effects or low bioavailability. Nonetheless, advances in biotechnology and synthetic biology are enabling scientists to produce these compounds more sustainably, often using engineered microbes to synthesize complex natural products.

    In recent years, **bioprospecting**—the search for medicinal compounds in nature—has gained momentum, with researchers looking to plants, marine life, and microorganisms for novel drugs. This approach combines traditional ethnobotanical knowledge with cutting-edge science, creating a new era of pharmacology that honors both ancient practices and modern innovation.

Conclusion

Modern pharmacology owes much of its success to natural compounds, which have served as the foundation for countless drugs that improve and save lives. By drawing inspiration from the natural world, pharmacologists have developed medications that address a wide range of health issues, from infectious diseases and chronic conditions to cancer and cardiovascular disorders. As research continues, the exploration of natural compounds remains a promising frontier in drug development, with the potential to yield new treatments and cures that harness the power of nature in combination with scientific advancements. This intersection of natural wisdom and modern science exemplifies the enduring value of natural compounds in the pursuit of better health and well-being.

Scientific Discoveries and Innovations: New Ways to Make Natural Remedies Safer and More Effective

Scientific discoveries and technological innovations are transforming the field of natural medicine, making traditional remedies safer, more effective, and easier to integrate into modern healthcare practices. By applying advanced techniques in research, extraction, formulation, and delivery, scientists are enhancing the therapeutic potential of natural remedies, ensuring consistent results and minimizing risks. These advances bridge the gap between age-old wisdom and contemporary medical standards, offering new and improved ways to harness the benefits of natural remedies.

1. **Advanced Extraction Techniques for Purity and Potency**

One of the most important innovations in natural medicine is the development of advanced extraction techniques that yield purer, more potent extracts with minimal impurities. Techniques such as **supercritical CO2 extraction, ultrasonic-assisted extraction**, and **microwave-assisted extraction** allow scientists to obtain high concentrations of active compounds from plants and herbs without using toxic solvents. Supercritical CO2 extraction, for example, uses pressurized carbon dioxide to extract essential oils and other compounds, resulting in highly pure and potent extracts ideal for therapeutic use. These methods provide greater control over the concentration and purity of natural remedies, making them safer and more effective.

2. Nanotechnology for Enhanced Absorption and Bioavailability

A significant challenge with many natural remedies is poor bioavailability, meaning the active compounds are not easily absorbed by the body. **Nanotechnology** offers a solution by creating nano-sized particles that improve the delivery and absorption of these compounds. For instance, **liposomal encapsulation** technology surrounds active ingredients with a lipid layer, allowing them to bypass the digestive system and be absorbed directly into the bloodstream. This approach has been particularly beneficial for curcumin (the active ingredient in turmeric), which has low natural bioavailability. Nanotechnology has increased curcumin's absorption, making it a more powerful anti-inflammatory and antioxidant agent. By enhancing bioavailability, nanotechnology ensures that natural remedies deliver their full therapeutic potential.

3. Standardization for Consistency and Reliability

Standardization has become a crucial innovation in the field of natural medicine, ensuring that each batch of a remedy contains a consistent level of active ingredients. In the past, the strength and potency of natural remedies could vary widely depending on factors like the plant's growing conditions, harvesting time, and preparation methods. Today, companies use standardized extracts, where the active compounds are measured and adjusted to meet a precise concentration. For example, standardized ginkgo biloba supplements contain a fixed percentage of flavonoids and terpenoids, ensuring that users receive the same potency with every dose. Standardization not only improves the reliability of natural remedies but also allows healthcare professionals to recommend precise dosages with confidence.

4. Targeted Delivery Systems for Focused Action

Modern innovations have also led to the development of targeted delivery systems, allowing natural remedies to act more effectively in specific areas of the body. **Enteric coating** is a technique used for remedies like probiotics, which need to reach the intestines to be effective. The coating protects the active ingredients from being destroyed by stomach acid, allowing them to reach their target location intact. Similarly, **time-release formulations** enable a gradual release of the active compound over several hours, providing sustained effects and reducing the need for multiple doses. These delivery systems enhance the effectiveness of natural remedies by ensuring they reach the areas where they are most needed.

5. Genetic and Biotechnological Advancements for Precision Medicine

Recent advancements in genetics and biotechnology have allowed scientists to explore the interaction between natural compounds and individual genetic profiles. With the rise of **personalized medicine**, it is now possible to tailor natural remedies to an individual's unique genetic makeup, increasing the likelihood of positive outcomes. For instance, genetic testing can identify individuals who may respond particularly well to specific herbal treatments or dietary supplements. Biotechnology is also being used to produce high-quality compounds through **plant cell culture** and **microbial fermentation**, ensuring a stable supply of rare ingredients without the need to harvest them from the environment.

6. Clinical Trials and Evidence-Based Validation

Another crucial development is the increased use of clinical trials to test the efficacy and safety of natural remedies. In the past, many natural remedies were used based on traditional knowledge and anecdotal evidence. Today, rigorous scientific studies are conducted to validate their effectiveness. Clinical trials help determine the appropriate dosage, identify potential side effects, and assess how these remedies interact with conventional medications. This evidence-based approach not only supports the integration of natural remedies into mainstream healthcare but also ensures that consumers have access to accurate and reliable information.

7. Artificial Intelligence for Accelerated Discovery

Artificial intelligence (AI) is now playing a role in accelerating the discovery of new natural remedies and understanding the mechanisms of known ones. AI algorithms can analyze vast amounts of data from scientific literature, traditional medicinal knowledge, and clinical trials to identify promising natural compounds and predict their effects on human health. By processing data quickly and efficiently, AI allows researchers to identify new therapeutic applications for natural remedies, optimize formulations, and even suggest potential synergies between natural compounds and pharmaceutical drugs. This technology is revolutionizing the research process, leading to faster and more targeted discoveries.

8 Sustainable Sourcing and Ethical Practices

With the growing demand for natural remedies, sustainable sourcing has become a priority in the field. Innovations in **sustainable agriculture**, **wild harvesting guidelines**, and **ethical trade practices** ensure that plants and other resources are harvested responsibly without depleting natural ecosystems. For example, endangered plants like certain species of ginseng are now grown in controlled environments rather than being harvested from the wild, ensuring a sustainable supply while protecting biodiversity. Sustainable sourcing practices not only support environmental health but also improve the quality and safety of natural remedies, as cultivated plants can be monitored for contaminants and grown under controlled conditions.

9. Quality Control and Safety Standards

Ensuring the safety of natural remedies has been greatly enhanced by improvements in quality control. Advances in **analytical chemistry** allow for precise testing of products to detect contaminants, such as heavy metals, pesticides, and microbial impurities. Techniques like **mass spectrometry** and **liquid chromatography** help verify the purity of natural products, ensuring they meet safety standards. These innovations in quality control are critical for consumer safety, as they help identify high-quality products and eliminate those that do not meet rigorous health and safety guidelines.

10. Synergistic Formulations for Enhanced Benefits

Another innovative approach involves creating synergistic formulations that combine multiple natural compounds to enhance their effects. Many active ingredients in natural remedies work better when used together, creating a synergy that amplifies their benefits. For instance, turmeric and black pepper are often combined because black pepper increases the bioavailability of curcumin, turmeric's active compound. Similarly, adaptogenic herbs like ashwagandha, rhodiola, and ginseng are often combined to provide a comprehensive approach to stress management. These formulations allow consumers to experience greater therapeutic effects from natural remedies without increasing the dosage of any single compound.

Chapter 3
Potent Medicinal Herbs and Plants
Examples of Traditional Plants (Turmeric, Echinacea, Ginseng) and Their Natural Benefits

Throughout history, various plants have been celebrated in traditional medicine systems for their health-enhancing properties. Today, many of these plants are still used and have gained scientific backing for their health benefits, making them popular choices in natural and integrative healthcare. Some of the most widely used and studied plants include **turmeric**, **echinacea**, and **ginseng**. Each of these plants offers unique compounds and therapeutic effects, showcasing the wisdom of ancient practices and their relevance in modern health.

1. Turmeric

Turmeric (*Curcuma longa*) is a bright yellow root that has been used for thousands of years in traditional Ayurvedic and Chinese medicine, primarily for its anti-inflammatory and antioxidant properties. The main active compound in turmeric, **curcumin**, is known for its ability to reduce inflammation and neutralize free radicals, protecting cells from oxidative damage. These properties make turmeric highly valuable in the management of chronic inflammatory conditions, such as arthritis and joint pain.

Modern research has confirmed many of turmeric's traditional uses and uncovered additional benefits. Curcumin has been found to support **heart health** by improving blood vessel function and reducing cholesterol levels. It may also play a role in **brain health**, as studies suggest curcumin can cross the blood-brain barrier, potentially reducing inflammation and oxidative damage in the brain. Additionally, curcumin's anti-inflammatory effects are believed to help with **digestive health** by reducing symptoms of conditions like irritable bowel syndrome (IBS). However, curcumin has low bioavailability on its own, which has led to the development of enhanced formulations, often combined with **piperine** from black pepper, to improve absorption.

2. Echinacea

Echinacea, commonly known as the purple coneflower, is a plant native to North America and has been used for centuries by Indigenous tribes for its immune-boosting properties. The plant contains bioactive compounds like **polysaccharides**, **flavonoids**, and **alkamides**, which work together to stimulate the immune system, making echinacea a popular remedy for preventing and managing colds and respiratory infections.

Studies have shown that echinacea can help **reduce the severity and duration of colds** by supporting white blood cell activity, which plays a critical role in defending the body against pathogens. In addition to its immune-boosting effects, echinacea has **anti-inflammatory** properties, which may benefit skin health, particularly in cases of mild acne or irritation. Echinacea is often taken as a supplement or in tea form and is frequently combined with other immune-supportive herbs, such as elderberry, during the cold and flu season. However, it is generally recommended to use echinacea intermittently or during the early stages of illness, as its effects are most potent when used as a short-term immune support.

3. Ginseng

Ginseng, particularly **Asian ginseng** (*Panax ginseng*) and **American ginseng** (*Panax quinquefolius*), is a prized medicinal herb in both traditional Chinese medicine and Native American healing practices. Known as an adaptogen, ginseng helps the body adapt to stress and supports overall vitality. The main active compounds in ginseng, called **ginsenosides**, have been found to influence the nervous, immune, and endocrine systems, providing a range of health benefits.

One of the most prominent uses of ginseng is for **energy and stamina**. Ginseng is believed to combat fatigue and increase mental alertness, making it a popular choice for those experiencing low energy or mental fatigue. Studies have also shown that ginseng can enhance **cognitive function**, improving memory and concentration, which has made it an appealing option for individuals seeking a natural way to boost mental performance.

Beyond energy and mental health, ginseng supports **immune function** by enhancing the activity of natural killer cells, which are crucial in defending the body against infections. Ginseng is also associated with **blood sugar regulation**, as some studies suggest that it may improve insulin sensitivity and help control blood glucose levels, making it beneficial for individuals managing type 2 diabetes. Additionally, ginseng has been linked to **sexual health** and is often used as a natural remedy for erectile dysfunction, particularly in Asian traditional medicine.

Summary of Benefits and Applications

Each of these plants—turmeric, echinacea, and ginseng—offers distinct health benefits rooted in centuries of traditional use and supported by modern research. Their roles in reducing inflammation, boosting the immune system, and enhancing physical and mental resilience make them valuable tools in natural and integrative healthcare. Whether used individually or as part of a holistic health regimen, these plants provide a natural, accessible means of supporting overall wellness.

Integrating Traditional Plants into Modern Healthcare

The popularity of these plants has led to a range of formulations, including capsules, tinctures, teas, and topical applications, making it easier for individuals to access their benefits. Thanks to ongoing scientific research and advances in formulation technology, traditional plants like turmeric, echinacea, and ginseng are more accessible, standardized, and effective than ever before, bridging the gap between ancient knowledge and contemporary health practices.

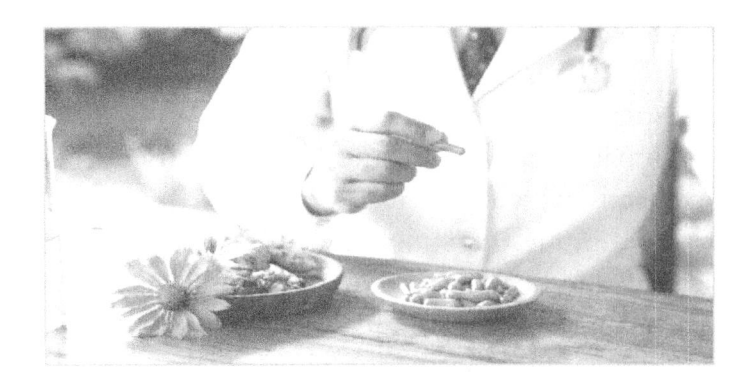

Each of these recipes features one or more of the beneficial plants discussed in this chapter: turmeric, echinacea and ginseng. These recipes offer not only delicious flavours, but also the healthy properties of these traditional ingredients.
Enhancing Health with Traditional Plants

25 beneficial recipes for general health

1. Golden Glow Latte
Description: A warm, anti-inflammatory drink that combines turmeric with black pepper for optimal absorption.
Ingredients:
1 cup almond milk (or any plant-based milk)
1/2 tsp **turmeric powder** (standardized to 95% curcuminoids) or 1 tsp freshly grated turmeric
1/4 tsp cinnamon (optional, for added flavor)
1/4 tsp ginger powder (optional, for digestive support)
A pinch of **black pepper** (to enhance curcumin absorption)
1 tsp honey or maple syrup (optional)
Instructions:
Heat almond milk in a saucepan until steaming.
Add turmeric, cinnamon, ginger, and black pepper. Whisk to combine.
Pour into a mug, add honey or maple syrup to taste, and serve warm.
Variations:
With Liposomal Curcumin: Substitute turmeric powder with 1/4 tsp liposomal curcumin for increased absorption. Omit black pepper if using this form.
Daily Use: Reduce turmeric to 1/4 tsp for daily anti-inflammatory support.
Nutritional Information: 90 kcal, 4g fat, 11g carbs, 1g protein

2. Immunity Elixir Tea
Description: Echinacea tea boosted with honey and lemon, perfect for immune support.
Ingredients:
1 echinacea tea bag
1 cup hot water
1 tsp honey
1/4 tsp lemon juice
Instructions:
Steep tea bag in hot water for 5 minutes.
Remove tea bag, stir in honey and lemon juice.
Variations:
Enhanced with Elderberry: Add 1 tsp elderberry syrup for added immune benefits.
Nutritional Information: 20 kcal, 0g fat, 5g carbs, 0g protein

3. Sunrise Energy Smoothie

Description: An energizing smoothie that combines turmeric and ginger for an anti-inflammatory boost.

Ingredients:
1 cup orange juice
1/2 tsp **turmeric powder**
1/4 tsp **ginger powder** or 1/2 tsp fresh ginger
1/2 banana
1 tbsp chia seeds

Instructions:
Blend all ingredients until smooth.
Pour into a glass and enjoy immediately.

Variations:
With Liposomal Curcumin: Replace turmeric powder with 1/4 tsp liposomal curcumin for better absorption.

Nutritional Information: 150 kcal, 3g fat, 33g carbs, 2g protein

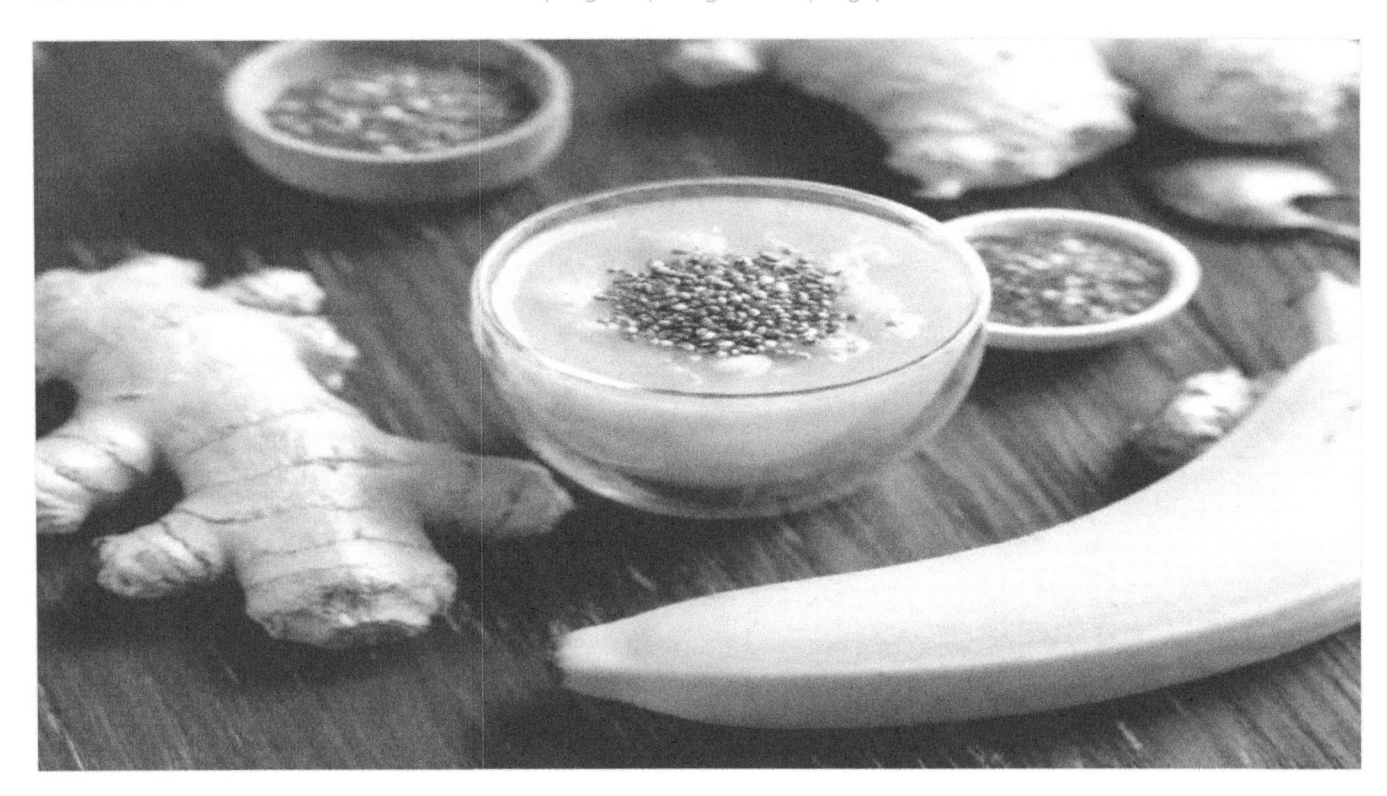

4. Citrus Vitality Cooler

Description: A refreshing drink with ginseng for energy and vitality.

Ingredients:
1 cup water
1/2 tsp **ginseng powder** (standardized for 10% ginsenosides)
1 tbsp lemon juice
1 tsp honey

Instructions:
Mix ginseng powder, lemon juice, and honey in a glass.
Add water, stir well, and serve over ice.

Variations:
Daily Use: Use 1/4 tsp ginseng for a milder effect.

Nutritional Information: 35 kcal, 0g fat, 9g carbs, 0g protein

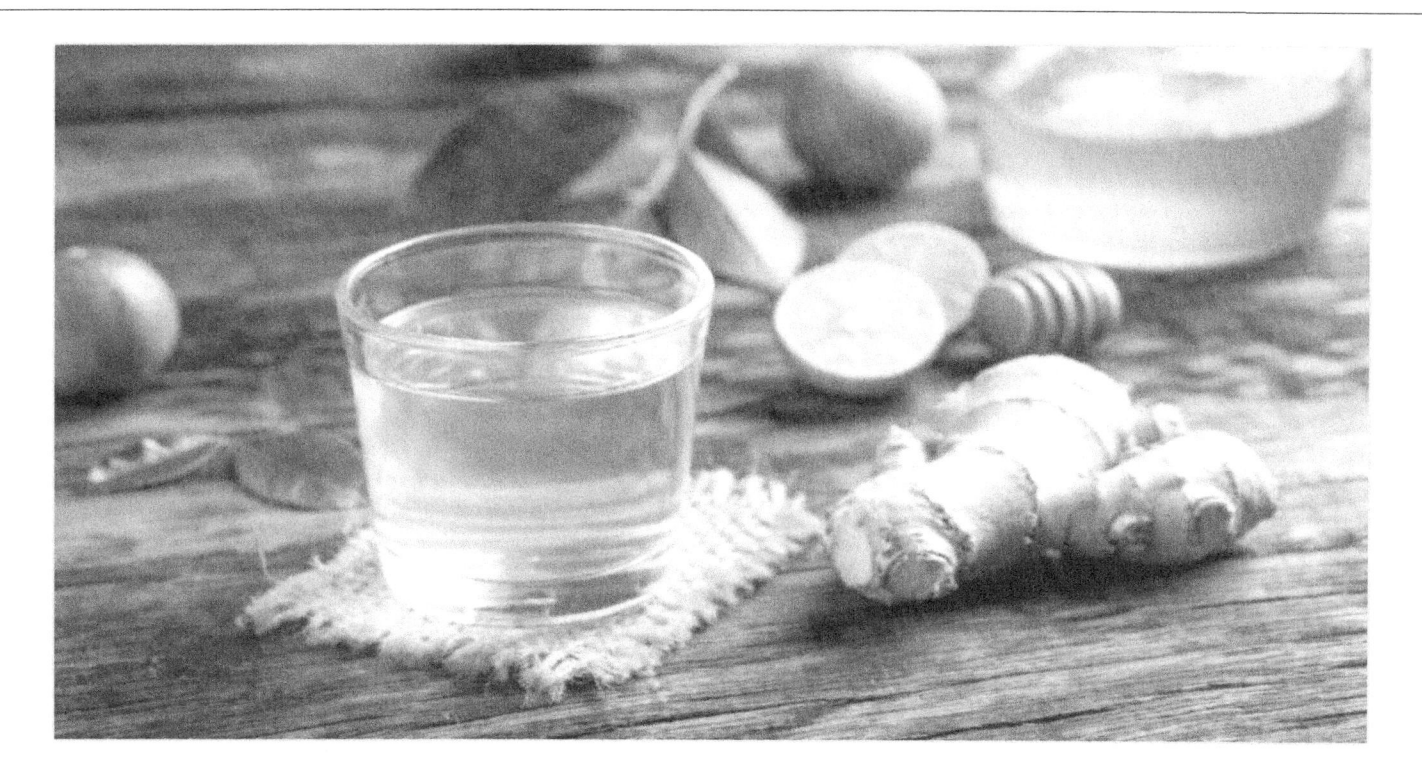

5. Spiced Turmeric Cauliflower Bites

Description: Roasted cauliflower with turmeric for a tasty anti-inflammatory side.
Ingredients:
2 cups cauliflower florets
1 tbsp olive oil
1/2 tsp **turmeric powder**
Salt and pepper to taste
Instructions:
Preheat oven to 400°F (200°C).
Toss cauliflower with olive oil, turmeric, salt, and pepper.
Spread on a baking sheet and roast for 25 minutes.
Variations:
Extra Spice: Add 1/4 tsp black pepper for enhanced curcumin absorption.
Nutritional Information: 120 kcal, 8g fat, 10g carbs, 2g protein

---

6. Herbal Lemonade Boost

Description: A cooling lemonade with echinacea for immune support.
Ingredients:
2 cups water
1 echinacea tea bag
1 tbsp lemon juice
1 tsp agave syrup
Instructions:
Steep tea bag in hot water for 5 minutes.
Chill, then add lemon juice and agave. Serve over ice.
Variations:
With Elderberry: Add 1 tsp elderberry extract for extra immune benefits.
Nutritional Information: 30 kcal, 0g fat, 8g carbs, 0g protein

7. Warm Cinnamon Ginseng Brew

Description: A warm drink with ginseng and cinnamon for energy and digestion.
Ingredients:
- 1 cup hot water
- 1/2 tsp **ginseng powder**
- 1/4 tsp cinnamon
- 1/2 tsp honey

Instructions:
Combine all ingredients in a mug.
Stir well and let steep for 5 minutes.

Variations:
With Ginger: Add 1/4 tsp ginger powder for extra digestive support.
Nutritional Information: 30 kcal, 0g fat, 7g carbs, 0g protein

---

8. Golden Honey-Glazed Carrots

Description: A sweet, turmeric-infused side dish.
Ingredients:
- 1 cup carrots, sliced
- 1 tsp honey
- 1/2 tsp **turmeric powder**
- 1 tsp olive oil

Instructions:
Preheat oven to 400°F (200°C).
Toss carrots with honey, turmeric, and olive oil.
Roast for 20 minutes or until tender.

Variations:
For Daily Use: Reduce turmeric to 1/4 tsp.
Nutritional Information: 80 kcal, 4g fat, 10g carbs, 1g protein

---

9. Ginger Power Tea

Description: Echinacea tea with ginger for an immune-boosting, warming drink.
Ingredients:
- 1 echinacea tea bag
- 1 cup hot water
- 1/2 tsp freshly grated ginger
- 1 tsp honey

Instructions:
Steep echinacea tea and ginger in hot water for 5 minutes.
Remove tea bag and stir in honey.

Variations:
Extra Immune Boost: Add a dash of lemon juice.
Nutritional Information: 25 kcal, 0g fat, 6g carbs, 0g protein

10. Green Energizer Smoothie

Description: A green smoothie with spinach, banana, and ginseng for mental clarity and energy.
Ingredients:
1 cup spinach
1/2 banana
1/2 tsp **ginseng powder**
1/2 cup almond milk
Instructions:
Blend all ingredients until smooth.
Pour into a glass and serve immediately.
Variations:
For Sustained Energy: Add 1 tsp chia seeds.
Nutritional Information: 60 kcal, 1g fat, 12g carbs, 2g protein

---

11. Sunshine Citrus Dressing

Description: A vibrant, anti-inflammatory turmeric dressing for salads.
Ingredients:
1/4 cup olive oil
1 tbsp lemon juice
1/2 tsp **turmeric powder**
1/4 tsp black pepper
Instructions:
Whisk ingredients together in a small bowl until combined.
Drizzle over your favorite salad.
Variations:
Enhanced Absorption: Use liposomal curcumin to replace turmeric powder.
Nutritional Information: 180 kcal, 18g fat, 2g carbs, 0g protein

---

12. Berry Immune-Boost Smoothie

Description: This smoothie is loaded with antioxidants from berries and includes echinacea for added immune support.
Ingredients:
1 cup mixed berries (strawberries, blueberries, blackberries)
1 echinacea tea bag, brewed and cooled
1/2 cup water
1 tsp honey
Instructions:
Brew echinacea tea and let it cool.
Add tea, berries, and honey to a blender and blend until smooth.
Variations:
Extra Vitamin C: Add 1/4 cup orange juice for an additional immune boost.
Nutritional Information: 100 kcal, 1g fat, 24g carbs, 1g protein

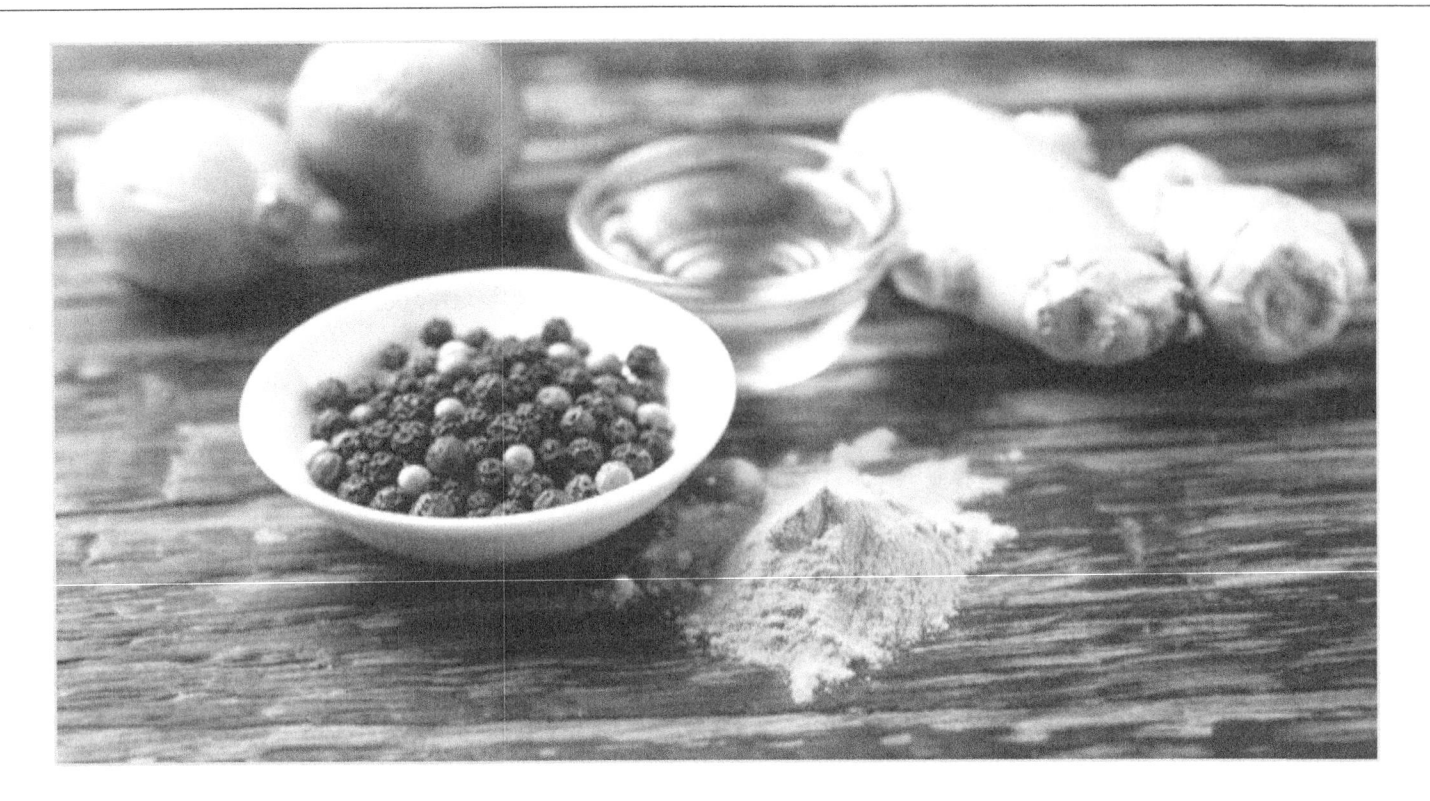

13. Turmeric Sunrise Oatmeal

Description: A warm, golden oatmeal with turmeric to start your day with an anti-inflammatory boost.

Ingredients:
1/2 cup rolled oats
1 cup water or almond milk
1/4 tsp **turmeric powder** (or 1/8 tsp liposomal curcumin)
1/2 tsp honey
A pinch of cinnamon (optional)

Instructions:
Bring water or almond milk to a boil, then add oats and turmeric.
Simmer until oats are tender, then stir in honey and cinnamon.

Variations:
Daily Use: Reduce turmeric to 1/8 tsp if using daily.
Nutritional Information: 120 kcal, 2g fat, 22g carbs, 4g protein

---

14. Ginseng Nutty Boost Smoothie

Description: A creamy smoothie with ginseng for energy, almond butter for protein, and banana for natural sweetness.

Ingredients:
1 cup almond milk
1/2 tsp **ginseng powder**
1 tsp almond butter
1/2 banana

Instructions:
Blend all ingredients together until smooth.
Serve immediately.

Variations:
Add Protein: Add 1 tbsp chia seeds for extra protein and fiber.
Nutritional Information: 160 kcal, 7g fat, 20g carbs, 3g protein

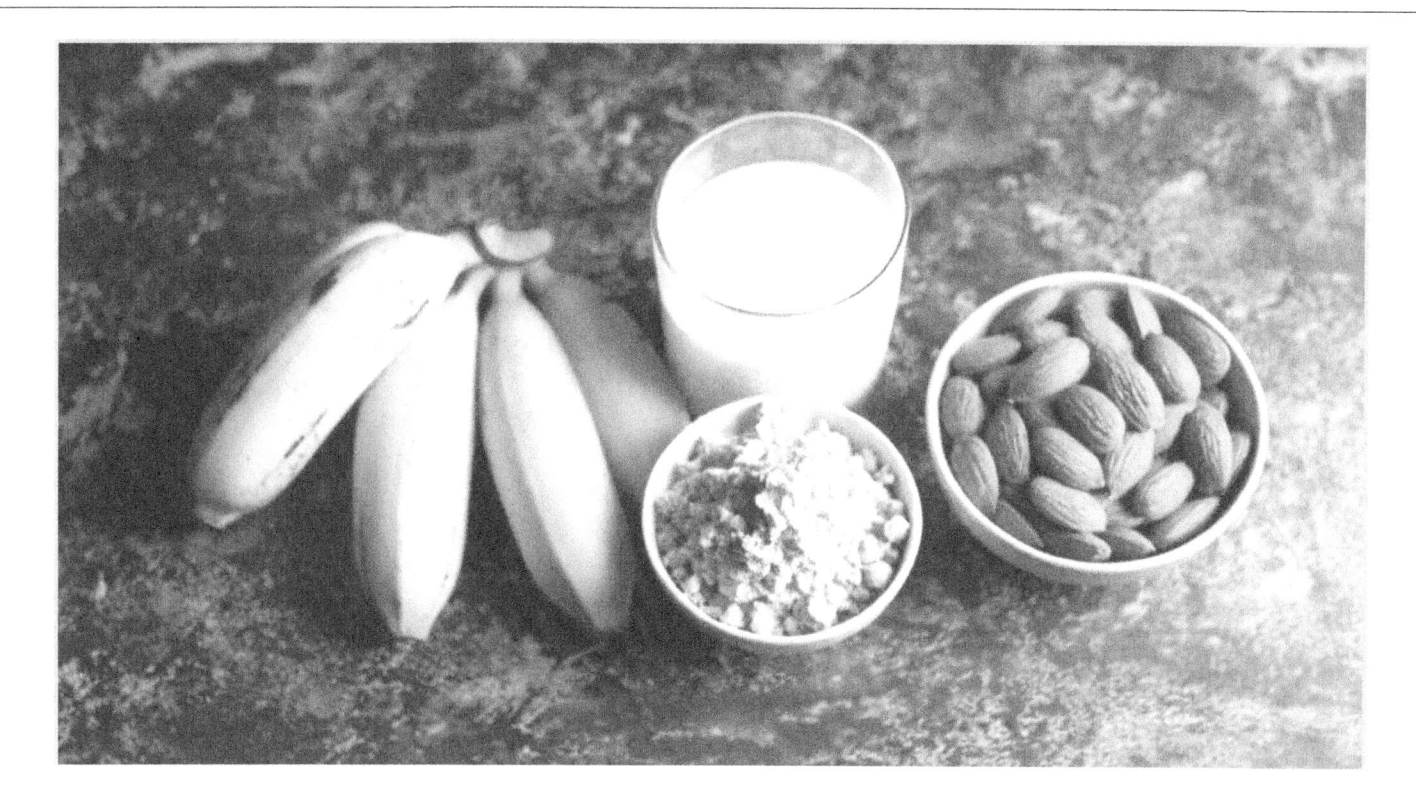

15. Golden Delight Hummus

Description: A vibrant, turmeric-infused hummus, ideal for dipping or spreading.
Ingredients:
1 cup cooked chickpeas
1/2 tsp **turmeric powder** (standardized to 95% curcuminoids)
1 tbsp olive oil
1 tbsp tahini
Salt, to taste
Instructions:
Blend all ingredients until smooth.
Adjust seasonings as desired and serve with vegetables or pita.
Variations:
Enhanced Absorption: Add a pinch of black pepper to improve curcumin bioavailability.
Nutritional Information: 150 kcal, 8g fat, 14g carbs, 4g protein

---

16. Apple Echinacea Cider

Description: A cozy, spiced apple cider with echinacea for added immune support.
Ingredients:
1 echinacea tea bag
1 cup apple cider
1/4 tsp cinnamon
Instructions:
Steep echinacea tea bag in hot apple cider for 5 minutes.
Stir in cinnamon and enjoy warm.
Variations:
For Extra Spice: Add a pinch of nutmeg or cloves.
Nutritional Information: 100 kcal, 0g fat, 25g carbs, 0g protein

17. Healing Turmeric Lentil Soup

Description: A hearty, anti-inflammatory soup with turmeric and lentils for a warming meal.

Ingredients:
1 cup dried lentils
1 tsp **turmeric powder**
1 clove garlic, minced
1/2 tsp cumin powder

Instructions:
Rinse lentils and add to a pot with 4 cups water, turmeric, garlic, and cumin.
Simmer until lentils are tender, about 20-25 minutes. Season with salt.

Variations:
Add Greens: Stir in spinach or kale for added nutrients.

Nutritional Information: 180 kcal, 1g fat, 32g carbs, 12g protein

---

18. Berry Bliss Compote

Description: A berry compote with ginseng, perfect as a topping for yogurt, pancakes, or oatmeal.

Ingredients:
1 cup mixed berries (fresh or frozen)
1/4 tsp **ginseng powder**
1 tbsp honey

Instructions:
Combine berries, ginseng powder, and honey in a saucepan.
Simmer over low heat until berries soften, about 10 minutes.

Variations:
With Extra Fiber: Add 1 tbsp chia seeds while simmering for a thicker consistency.

Nutritional Information: 70 kcal, 0g fat, 18g carbs, 1g protein

---

19. Detox Sunshine Water

Description: A refreshing detox drink with turmeric and lemon to support digestion and hydration.

Ingredients:
1 liter water
1 tsp **turmeric powder** or 1/4 tsp liposomal curcumin
1 lemon, sliced

Instructions:
Combine water, turmeric, and lemon slices in a pitcher.
Let sit for at least 10 minutes before drinking.

Variations:
With Fresh Herbs: Add mint or basil for extra flavor.

Nutritional Information: 5 kcal, 0g fat, 1g carbs, 0g protein

20. Iced Mint Echinacea Tea

Description: A refreshing, immune-supportive iced tea with echinacea and fresh mint.
Ingredients:
1 echinacea tea bag
1 cup water
1 sprig fresh mint
Ice
Instructions:
Brew echinacea tea, let it cool, and pour over ice.
Garnish with fresh mint.
Variations:
Add Lemon: Add a slice of lemon for extra immune support.
Nutritional Information: 5 kcal, 0g fat, 1g carbs, 0g protein

21. Golden Herb Pilaf

Description: A fragrant rice pilaf with turmeric for anti-inflammatory benefits.
Ingredients:
1 cup rice
1/2 tsp **turmeric powder**
1 tbsp olive oil
Salt, to taste
Instructions:
Heat olive oil in a pan, add rice and turmeric, stirring to coat.
Add water according to package instructions and cook until tender.
Variations:
With Extra Spice: Add 1/4 tsp black pepper for improved curcumin absorption.
Nutritional Information: 180 kcal, 5g fat, 30g carbs, 3g protein

22. Calm and Sleep Tea Blend

Description: A calming blend of echinacea and chamomile, ideal before bedtime.
Ingredients:
1 echinacea tea bag
1 chamomile tea bag
1 cup hot water
Instructions:
Steep both tea bags in hot water for 5-7 minutes.
Remove tea bags and enjoy warm.
Variations:
Add Honey: Add 1 tsp honey for natural sweetness and calming effects.
Nutritional Information: 5 kcal, 0g fat, 1g carbs, 0g protein

23. Golden Avocado Toast

Description: Avocado toast with turmeric for a nutrient-packed, anti-inflammatory boost.
Ingredients:
1 slice whole-grain bread, toasted
1/2 avocado, mashed
1/4 tsp **turmeric powder**
Salt and pepper, to taste
Instructions:
Spread mashed avocado on toast, sprinkle with turmeric, salt, and pepper.
Serve immediately.
Variations:
For Enhanced Absorption: Add a pinch of black pepper.
Nutritional Information: 150 kcal, 8g fat, 15g carbs, 3g protein

24. Turmeric & Citrus Detox Salad

Description: A refreshing salad combining the anti-inflammatory benefits of turmeric with the cleansing properties of citrus, ideal for supporting digestion and detoxification.
Ingredients:
1 cup mixed greens (such as spinach, arugula, or kale)
1/2 orange, segmented
1/4 avocado, sliced
1/2 tsp **turmeric powder** (or 1/4 tsp liposomal curcumin for better absorption)
1 tbsp lemon juice
1 tbsp olive oil
Salt and pepper to taste
Instructions:
Arrange mixed greens, orange segments, and avocado slices on a plate.
In a small bowl, whisk together turmeric powder, lemon juice, olive oil, salt, and pepper.
Drizzle dressing over the salad and toss gently to combine.
Variations:
Enhanced Absorption: Use 1/4 tsp liposomal curcumin in the dressing and omit black pepper.
Extra Flavor: Add 1/2 tsp grated ginger to the dressing for an additional digestive boost.
Nutritional Information: 170 kcal, 12g fat, 15g carbs, 2g protein

25. Spicy Ginseng Ginger Shots

Description: A potent shot that combines the energizing effects of ginseng with the anti-inflammatory benefits of ginger, perfect for a quick pick-me-up.
Ingredients:
1/2 tsp **ginseng powder** (standardized to 10% ginsenosides)
1/2 tsp freshly grated ginger or 1/4 tsp ginger powder
1 tbsp lemon juice
1/4 cup water
1/2 tsp honey (optional, for sweetness)
Instructions:
In a small blender, combine ginseng powder, ginger, lemon juice, water, and honey.
Blend until smooth. If desired, strain the mixture for a smoother texture.
Pour into a small glass and drink immediately.
Variations:
For Milder Flavor: Reduce ginseng to 1/4 tsp for a gentler energy boost.
Enhanced Absorption: Add a pinch of black pepper to enhance ginger's absorption.
Nutritional Information: 15 kcal, 0g fat, 3g carbs, 0g protein

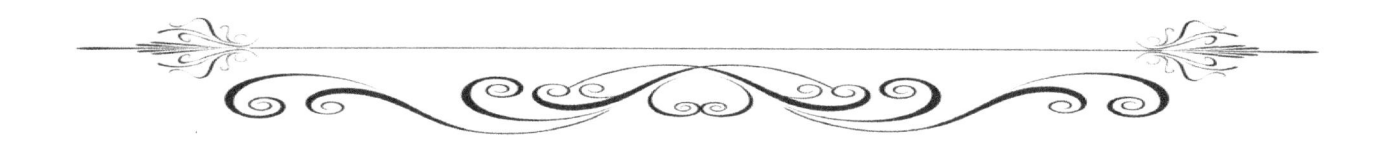

Chapter 4

Integrative Approaches to Well-being

Combating Inflammation and Pain: The Use of Natural Remedies Like Devil's Claw and Modern Techniques to Enhance Relief

Inflammation is a natural response of the immune system to protect the body from infections, injuries, or toxins. However, chronic inflammation is linked to numerous health issues, including arthritis, cardiovascular diseases, and autoimmune disorders. Pain, often associated with inflammation, can be a significant barrier to daily functioning and quality of life. Natural remedies, such as **Devil's Claw** (*Harpagophytum procumbens*), turmeric, and ginger, have long been used to manage inflammation and pain. When combined with modern techniques like targeted delivery systems and scientific formulations, these remedies offer an effective, holistic approach to managing inflammation and providing pain relief.

Understanding Devil's Claw and Its Benefits

Devil's Claw, a plant native to southern Africa, has a long history in traditional medicine for treating pain and inflammation. Its name comes from the claw-like shape of its fruit, but the medicinal power lies in its root. The primary active compounds in Devil's Claw are **harpagosides**, which have been shown to possess anti-inflammatory and analgesic properties. These compounds work by inhibiting pathways that lead to inflammation and pain, similar to how nonsteroidal anti-inflammatory drugs (NSAIDs) work but with fewer side effects.

Research suggests that Devil's Claw can help reduce symptoms in conditions such as:

Osteoarthritis: Studies show that Devil's Claw can help alleviate joint pain, making it easier for people with osteoarthritis to improve mobility.

Lower Back Pain: Devil's Claw has been found effective in reducing chronic lower back pain, often associated with inflammation and muscle strain.

Rheumatic Diseases: The anti-inflammatory effects of Devil's Claw make it beneficial in managing symptoms of other inflammatory diseases like rheumatoid arthritis.

Other Natural Remedies for Inflammation and Pain

While Devil's Claw is a popular natural remedy for pain, it is not the only effective option. There are several other herbs and natural compounds known for their anti-inflammatory and pain-relieving properties:

Turmeric (Curcuma longa): Turmeric contains curcumin, a powerful anti-inflammatory compound. Studies have shown that curcumin reduces inflammatory markers in the body and can be as effective as some NSAIDs in alleviating pain, especially in arthritis. However, curcumin has low bioavailability, so combining it with black pepper or using formulations with enhanced absorption can increase its effectiveness.

Ginger (Zingiber officinale): Ginger has been used in traditional medicine for thousands of years to treat inflammation and pain. It contains gingerols, which have anti-inflammatory and antioxidant properties. Ginger can reduce pain in osteoarthritis and may also help in managing muscle pain from exercise.

Boswellia (Boswellia serrata): Also known as Indian frankincense, Boswellia contains boswellic acids that have strong anti-inflammatory effects. Boswellia is often used in the treatment of inflammatory conditions like arthritis and has been found to help in reducing joint swelling and improving mobility.

Willow Bark (Salix alba): Known as nature's aspirin, willow bark contains salicin, a compound similar to aspirin, which provides pain relief. It is commonly used to alleviate headaches, lower back pain, and osteoarthritis pain.

Capsaicin: Derived from chili peppers, capsaicin is commonly used in topical creams to provide pain relief. It works by depleting a neurotransmitter called substance P, which transmits pain signals to the brain.

Modern Techniques to Enhance the Effectiveness of Natural Remedies

The efficacy of natural remedies can be further amplified by combining traditional wisdom with modern scientific advancements. Here are some of the ways modern techniques improve the effectiveness of these remedies:

1. Advanced Extraction and Standardization

To ensure consistency and potency, modern techniques are used to extract active compounds from natural remedies in their purest form. For instance, **standardized extracts** of Devil's Claw ensure a specific amount of harpagosides per dose, providing predictable and reliable results. This process also allows for safer, more potent formulations that retain the beneficial properties of the natural plant without unwanted contaminants.

2. Enhanced Bioavailability

Bioavailability—the rate and extent to which active compounds are absorbed into the bloodstream—is a significant challenge with many natural remedies. Compounds like curcumin in turmeric have low bioavailability, meaning that the body absorbs only a small amount of it. To improve this, modern formulations use techniques like **liposomal encapsulation, nanoemulsion**, and **piperine (black pepper extract)** to enhance absorption. These innovations allow the active ingredients to remain in the bloodstream longer, making them more effective in managing pain and inflammation.

3. Targeted Delivery Systems

Topical applications like creams, gels, and patches allow for **localized pain relief** by delivering active compounds directly to the affected area. For example, capsaicin and menthol are often included in topical creams for joint pain relief, and transdermal patches with Devil's Claw or Boswellia extracts can provide continuous, targeted relief. These applications reduce systemic absorption, minimizing the risk of side effects.

4. Synergistic Formulations

Research has shown that combining certain natural compounds can produce a **synergistic effect**, enhancing their effectiveness. For example, combining curcumin from turmeric with

Boswellia has been shown to improve pain and inflammation more than either ingredient alone. Formulations that incorporate Devil's Claw with turmeric or ginger can also provide a broader spectrum of relief for joint and muscle pain. By targeting multiple inflammatory pathways, these synergistic formulas offer more comprehensive pain relief.

5. Clinical Trials and Evidence-Based Dosing
Modern clinical trials help establish effective dosing guidelines for natural remedies, which were traditionally used based on empirical knowledge. These trials have verified the efficacy of natural remedies like Devil's Claw, turmeric, and Boswellia, allowing healthcare providers to recommend precise doses for conditions like arthritis, back pain, and other inflammatory disorders. With more research, the standardization of doses for specific conditions continues to improve, providing users with effective and safe natural options for pain relief.

Integrating Natural Remedies with Conventional Treatments
For those who experience chronic pain or inflammation, integrating natural remedies with conventional treatments can provide a more balanced approach to pain management. Many individuals find that using Devil's Claw or turmeric supplements alongside physical therapy, acupuncture, or even NSAIDs allows them to manage symptoms more effectively and with fewer side effects. For instance, a person with osteoarthritis might use a daily supplement of Boswellia and Devil's Claw to reduce joint inflammation, while applying a capsaicin cream directly to affected joints for additional relief.

Practical Considerations and Safety
While natural remedies are generally safer than pharmaceuticals, it is still essential to use them responsibly:
Consultation with Healthcare Providers: Individuals with chronic pain or inflammatory conditions should consult a healthcare provider before starting any natural remedy, especially if they are taking other medications. Some natural compounds can interact with prescription drugs.
Allergies and Sensitivities: Always check for allergies to plant-based compounds, as some individuals may be sensitive to ingredients like salicin in willow bark or ginger.
Dosage and Duration: Natural remedies are most effective when used as directed. Overuse can lead to adverse effects, such as gastrointestinal upset with excessive ginger or blood-thinning effects with high doses of turmeric.

By combining traditional remedies like Devil's Claw, turmeric, and ginger with modern advancements in formulation and delivery, we have access to a powerful, holistic approach to managing inflammation and pain. This synergy between ancient knowledge and scientific innovation allows individuals to find relief while minimizing the need for synthetic drugs, supporting a balanced approach to health and wellness. With continued research, the role of natural remedies in pain management is becoming increasingly validated, offering hope and relief to those seeking alternative options for a healthier, pain-free life.

Dosage and Modern Variants: Utilizing Advanced Extraction Methods and Optimized Dosing
The effectiveness of natural remedies has been greatly enhanced by advancements in extraction methods and optimized dosing. Traditional uses of plants and herbs relied on

variable doses, often dictated by availability or empirical knowledge passed down through generations. Today, however, modern science has refined the ways we extract and dose natural compounds, allowing for more consistent, potent, and safe applications. These innovations ensure that active ingredients are delivered in precise, therapeutic doses, maximizing their efficacy while reducing the risk of side effects.

Optimized Extraction Methods for Consistency and Potency

One of the biggest challenges with natural remedies is ensuring consistency in the concentration of active compounds. The potency of herbal extracts can vary widely depending on factors such as the season, geographical location, and growing conditions of the plant. Modern extraction techniques, however, allow scientists to isolate and concentrate these active compounds in controlled environments, resulting in more predictable and reliable formulations.

Supercritical CO_2 Extraction: This advanced method uses carbon dioxide under high pressure to extract essential compounds without using chemical solvents. The process is particularly effective for heat-sensitive compounds found in plants, such as curcumin from turmeric and gingerols from ginger. Supercritical CO_2 extraction yields a pure, highly concentrated product that maintains the integrity of the natural compounds.

Ultrasonic-Assisted Extraction: Ultrasonic waves break down plant cell walls, releasing the active compounds more effectively. This technique requires less time and lower temperatures, preserving the potency of delicate compounds and yielding extracts with high bioavailability. Ultrasonic extraction is commonly used for compounds like harpagosides in Devil's Claw, ensuring consistent potency in the final product.

Standardized Extracts: Standardization is the process of ensuring each dose contains a specific amount of active compounds. For example, standardized extracts of turmeric contain a precise percentage of curcuminoids, while Devil's Claw supplements often specify a harpagoside concentration. This level of precision allows healthcare providers and users to rely on consistent dosages, enhancing both the safety and efficacy of the remedy.

Liposomal Encapsulation: Liposomal technology involves encapsulating active compounds in tiny lipid bubbles called liposomes. This technique increases the bioavailability of compounds like curcumin, which are naturally difficult for the body to absorb. Liposomal encapsulation ensures that the active ingredients are absorbed more effectively, allowing for lower doses with higher effectiveness.

Tinctures and Liquid Extracts: These forms are created through alcohol or glycerin extraction and allow for easy, adjustable dosing. Tinctures are particularly popular in herbal medicine because they allow the active compounds to be quickly absorbed into the bloodstream. Liquid extracts of Devil's Claw, ginger, and turmeric can be precisely measured, providing flexibility in dosing and convenient administration for users who prefer not to take capsules or tablets.

Optimized Dosage for Maximum Effectiveness

Determining the correct dosage is essential for natural remedies to achieve therapeutic benefits without adverse effects. Modern research has helped establish standardized dosages that are both safe and effective for specific health conditions. Here's how optimized dosing is achieved in popular anti-inflammatory and pain-relief remedies:

Turmeric/Curcumin: Curcumin, the active compound in turmeric, has been studied extensively, and research indicates that it can be effective in doses of 500–2,000 mg per day. When taken as a supplement, curcumin is often combined with piperine (black pepper extract) or delivered in a liposomal form to enhance absorption. These optimized formulations allow for lower doses that are more effective and avoid the need to consume large quantities of raw turmeric.

Devil's Claw (Harpagophytum procumbens): The recommended dose of Devil's Claw is typically standardized to 50–100 mg of harpagosides per day. This optimized dosage has been shown to reduce pain and improve mobility in conditions like osteoarthritis. Modern extracts provide a concentrated form of harpagosides, ensuring that users receive the full therapeutic benefits without needing to take excessive amounts.

Ginger: Ginger is used in doses of 500–1,500 mg per day, depending on the intended use. For example, lower doses are effective for digestive support, while higher doses are beneficial for managing inflammation and muscle pain. Modern formulations often provide gingerol-standardized extracts, making it easier to achieve consistent results with lower doses.

Boswellia (Boswellia serrata): Commonly used for inflammatory conditions like arthritis, the recommended dose for Boswellia is typically 300–500 mg per day standardized to contain 60–65% boswellic acids. New extraction techniques help maintain high levels of these active compounds, making it possible to achieve effective anti-inflammatory results with minimal intake.

Willow Bark: Willow bark, often referred to as "nature's aspirin," provides natural pain relief. The standard dosage is generally 240 mg of salicin per day, the equivalent of a low-dose aspirin. Standardized extracts ensure consistent pain relief while reducing the risk of gastrointestinal issues often associated with synthetic aspirin.

Customized Formulations and Delivery Methods

Modern extraction methods and optimized doses are further complemented by **customized formulations and delivery methods** tailored to different needs and preferences:

Capsules and Tablets: These are the most common forms of natural remedy supplements, allowing for precise, standardized dosing and convenient storage. Many capsules contain enhanced extracts or combinations with bioavailability enhancers, such as curcumin with piperine.

Topical Creams and Gels: For conditions like joint pain, topical formulations provide targeted relief by delivering active ingredients directly to the affected area. Devil's Claw, Boswellia, and capsaicin are often included in topical products that reduce localized inflammation and pain without systemic effects.

Effervescent Tablets and Powders: These dissolvable forms are convenient for individuals who have difficulty swallowing pills and allow for quick absorption. Effervescent turmeric or ginger powders, for example, can be mixed with water for an easy-to-drink anti-inflammatory boost.

The Role of Modern Research in Dosing Precision
With increased scientific research into the pharmacokinetics of natural compounds, modern medicine has been able to fine-tune dosages for maximum effectiveness and safety. Clinical studies provide evidence-based guidelines for dosing, ensuring that users receive the therapeutic benefits of these natural remedies with minimal risk of side effects. For instance, research has shown that high doses of certain compounds, like curcumin or ginger, may cause digestive upset, guiding manufacturers to adjust dosages or recommend taking supplements with meals.

Studies also allow for the development of **condition-specific dosages**. For example:

Arthritis: Devil's Claw and turmeric are often dosed at higher levels for anti-inflammatory effects, whereas smaller doses may suffice for general wellness.

Digestive Health: Ginger and turmeric are commonly used in lower doses for daily digestive support, with adjustments based on individual tolerance.

Safety and Precision: Ensuring Effective Natural Remedies

Advanced extraction methods and optimized dosing have made it possible to harness the therapeutic potential of natural remedies more effectively and safely than ever before. By providing standardized, potent doses, these innovations allow users to incorporate natural remedies into their healthcare routines with confidence. Furthermore, modern research continues to refine dosing guidelines, making it easier for healthcare providers to recommend natural remedies alongside conventional treatments, ensuring a balanced, integrative approach to health and wellness.

In conclusion, the optimized extraction and dosing of natural remedies offer a bridge between ancient wisdom and modern science, making these natural therapies more accessible, effective, and safe. With continued advancements in extraction technology and dosing research, the future of natural remedies looks promising, as they become a reliable complement to conventional medicine in managing inflammation, pain, and other health conditions.

Mental Health and Stress: Ancient Remedies for Calm and Sleep (Like Chamomile and Lavender) with the Support of Modern Techniques Like Biofeedback and Mindfulness

In today's fast-paced world, mental health challenges and stress-related issues are common, affecting both quality of life and physical well-being. While modern medicine offers various treatments for stress and anxiety, ancient remedies such as **chamomile** and **lavender** have been used for centuries to promote relaxation and sleep. These gentle, plant-based solutions are now increasingly complemented by modern techniques, such as **biofeedback** and **mindfulness**, which empower individuals to manage stress more effectively. Together, these approaches create a balanced and holistic framework for supporting mental well-being, relaxation, and sleep.

Ancient Remedies for Calm and Sleep
For centuries, people have turned to plants like chamomile and lavender to soothe anxiety, improve sleep, and promote a sense of calm. These natural remedies work by affecting the body's nervous system, helping it transition from a state of alertness to one of relaxation.
Chamomile (Matricaria chamomilla): Chamomile is one of the oldest and most widely used herbal remedies for promoting relaxation and sleep. It contains an active compound called **apigenin**, which binds to receptors in the brain that help reduce anxiety and initiate sleep. Chamomile is commonly consumed as a tea before bedtime, but it is also available in capsule or tincture form for more precise dosing. Research has shown that chamomile can help reduce symptoms of mild anxiety and promote deeper, more restful sleep, making it ideal for those struggling with insomnia or general restlessness.
Lavender (Lavandula angustifolia): Known for its calming fragrance, lavender has long been used in aromatherapy to promote relaxation and alleviate stress. Lavender contains compounds like **linalool** and **linalyl acetate**, which interact with the brain to produce calming effects. Studies have shown that lavender can reduce symptoms of anxiety, improve mood, and even lower blood pressure and heart rate. Lavender essential oil can be diffused in the air, added to a warm bath, or applied topically to help calm the mind and prepare the body for sleep. In some cases, it is also taken orally in capsule form to reduce anxiety symptoms.
Valerian Root (Valeriana officinalis): Valerian root has been used as a sleep aid and anxiety remedy for hundreds of years. It contains compounds that enhance **gamma-aminobutyric acid (GABA)** in the brain, a neurotransmitter that promotes relaxation. Valerian is commonly taken as a tea or in supplement form and can be especially helpful for individuals experiencing sleeplessness due to anxiety.

Modern Techniques to Enhance Mental Health and Manage Stress
While natural remedies offer gentle, effective ways to address stress and support sleep, modern techniques such as biofeedback and mindfulness practices can further enhance these effects. These approaches provide individuals with tools to manage stress proactively and create long-term improvements in mental well-being.
Biofeedback: Biofeedback is a technique that uses electronic monitoring to help individuals become aware of physiological processes like heart rate, muscle tension, and breathing. By observing these processes, people can learn to control their stress response more effectively. For example, biofeedback can help individuals practice **deep breathing** or **progressive muscle relaxation**, which are both effective at lowering stress levels. When combined with calming herbs like chamomile or lavender, biofeedback can amplify the effects of these remedies by helping people achieve a state of deep relaxation more quickly and consistently.
Mindfulness and Meditation: Mindfulness practices involve focusing attention on the present moment, which helps reduce stress and promote a sense of calm. Techniques such as **mindful breathing**, **body scan meditations**, and **guided imagery** encourage individuals to observe their thoughts and sensations without judgment, reducing feelings of anxiety. When used alongside herbal remedies like lavender, mindfulness and meditation practices can enhance relaxation, making it easier to transition into restful sleep.
Cognitive Behavioral Therapy for Insomnia (CBT-I): CBT-I is a structured program that helps individuals address thoughts and behaviors that interfere with sleep. This approach can

be paired with natural remedies, such as chamomile tea or valerian supplements, to create a dual approach to managing insomnia. By retraining the brain's response to sleep-related cues, CBT-I helps individuals fall asleep more easily and enjoy higher-quality rest.

Breathwork and Relaxation Techniques: Techniques like **4-7-8 breathing** (inhale for 4 seconds, hold for 7, and exhale for 8) can activate the body's relaxation response and reduce stress quickly. These techniques, when practiced consistently, make the nervous system more resilient to stress. Combined with chamomile or lavender before bedtime, these breathing exercises can deepen relaxation, preparing both mind and body for rest.

Integrating Ancient Remedies and Modern Techniques for Comprehensive Stress Relief

Using ancient remedies together with modern techniques offers a comprehensive approach to managing stress and supporting mental health. Here are some practical ways to integrate these methods:

Chamomile Tea with Evening Meditation: Drinking chamomile tea an hour before bed, followed by a guided meditation or mindful breathing exercise, can create a powerful routine for relaxation. This combination encourages the nervous system to shift into a calm, restful state, reducing the likelihood of anxiety or racing thoughts at bedtime.

Lavender Aromatherapy with Biofeedback Sessions: Lavender essential oil can be diffused in the room or applied topically during biofeedback sessions to enhance relaxation. The scent of lavender can naturally lower blood pressure and heart rate, complementing the effects of biofeedback training.

Valerian Root Supplement with CBT-I Techniques: For individuals experiencing chronic insomnia, taking valerian root supplements alongside CBT-I practices can help break the cycle of sleeplessness and anxiety. The calming effects of valerian root make it easier to fall asleep, while CBT-I techniques help reframe negative associations with sleep, creating a sustainable approach to better rest.

Lavender Pillow Spray and Body Scan Meditation: Spraying a lavender mist on your pillow before bed and practicing a body scan meditation (mentally scanning and relaxing each part of the body) can be an effective way to transition into sleep. The soothing properties of lavender combined with the mindful attention of a body scan help to calm the mind and relax the body.

Practical Tips for Using Ancient Remedies and Techniques Together

To maximize the benefits of these combined approaches, consider the following tips:

Consistency Is Key: Regular use of herbal remedies and mindfulness practices helps to train the body and mind to respond to stress in a calmer, more adaptive way. Aim to establish a daily or nightly routine that incorporates your chosen remedy and relaxation technique.

Start Small and Adjust: Begin with small doses of chamomile, lavender, or valerian, and incorporate one relaxation technique at a time. Gradually increase your use of both remedies and techniques based on your comfort level and response.

Personalize Your Routine: Each person responds differently to various remedies and techniques. Experiment to find the combination that best supports your relaxation and sleep goals, and make adjustments as needed.

Incorporating both ancient and modern approaches to managing stress and supporting mental health creates a well-rounded, sustainable strategy for well-being. Herbal remedies like chamomile, lavender, and valerian offer natural solutions for relaxation and sleep, while techniques like biofeedback, mindfulness, and CBT-I provide additional tools to manage stress more effectively. Together, these practices empower individuals to take control of their mental health and cultivate a calmer, more resilient approach to life. By blending the wisdom of traditional healing with the precision of modern science, it's possible to achieve a state of balance that supports long-term mental and emotional health.

Digestion and Immunity: Traditional Uses of Natural Probiotics, Supported and Enhanced by Modern Science

The health of our digestive system is intricately linked to our immune system, as nearly 70% of immune cells reside in the gut. For centuries, various cultures around the world have turned to **natural probiotics** to promote gut health and bolster immunity, using fermented foods like yogurt, sauerkraut, and kimchi. These foods contain beneficial bacteria that support a balanced gut microbiome, enhancing both digestion and immunity. Modern science has validated and expanded on the benefits of these traditional practices, identifying specific probiotic strains and refining ways to deliver probiotics more effectively, making them a cornerstone of both digestive and immune health.

Traditional Uses of Natural Probiotics

Long before probiotics became a popular health trend, traditional diets around the world incorporated fermented foods as a primary source of beneficial bacteria. These foods not only preserved nutrients but also provided essential support for the digestive system and immune function.

Yogurt: Perhaps the most widely recognized natural probiotic, yogurt has been consumed for thousands of years in many cultures. Yogurt is made by fermenting milk with lactic acid bacteria, primarily **Lactobacillus** and **Bifidobacterium** strains, which promote a healthy gut environment. Regular consumption of yogurt has been shown to improve lactose digestion, regulate bowel movements, and support immune function.

Sauerkraut: Fermented cabbage, or sauerkraut, is a staple in many European cultures. Rich in **Lactobacillus** bacteria, sauerkraut not only aids digestion but also provides immune-boosting vitamins like vitamin C. Traditionally, sauerkraut was used to support gut health and prevent digestive issues, especially during winter months when fresh vegetables were scarce.

Kimchi: A Korean staple, kimchi is a spicy, fermented vegetable dish that contains a variety of probiotics, including **Lactobacillus plantarum**. Kimchi is known for supporting digestion, improving nutrient absorption, and enhancing immune defenses due to its rich probiotic content and antioxidants. Its combination of spices, garlic, and ginger also adds antimicrobial benefits, helping to protect the gut from harmful pathogens.

Kefir: Originating from the Caucasus region, kefir is a fermented milk drink that contains a more diverse range of beneficial bacteria and yeast than yogurt. The probiotics in kefir, particularly **Lactobacillus kefiri**, are effective at colonizing the gut and supporting both digestion and immunity. Kefir has been traditionally used to improve digestion, reduce inflammation, and enhance the body's natural defenses.

Miso and Natto: In Japan, fermented soy products like miso and natto have been staples for centuries. Miso soup, made from fermented soybeans, provides beneficial bacteria along with digestive enzymes, which help the body break down food more effectively. Natto, a fermented soybean dish rich in **Bacillus subtilis**, is known for its immune-enhancing properties and benefits for heart health.

The Science Behind Probiotics and Their Role in Digestive and Immune Health

Modern science has confirmed and expanded upon the traditional knowledge of fermented foods, revealing the specific mechanisms through which probiotics benefit the body. Probiotics are now recognized as a crucial factor in maintaining a balanced gut microbiome, a diverse community of bacteria that plays a key role in digestion, immune function, and even mental health.

Gut Health and Digestion: Probiotics support digestion by breaking down food and aiding in the absorption of nutrients, such as vitamins and minerals. Specific probiotic strains, such as **Lactobacillus rhamnosus** and **Bifidobacterium lactis**, produce enzymes that help digest lactose and other difficult-to-digest sugars. They also help maintain a balanced gut environment, reducing bloating, gas, and irregular bowel movements.

Immune System Support: The gut is a key player in immune health, as it contains specialized immune cells that respond to harmful pathogens. Probiotics help strengthen the immune system by stimulating the production of protective antibodies, promoting a balanced immune response, and preventing the overgrowth of harmful bacteria. **Lactobacillus casei** and **Bifidobacterium bifidum** are two strains shown to reduce the severity and frequency of respiratory infections and boost overall immunity.

Prevention of Gastrointestinal Infections: Probiotics help protect the gut lining from infections caused by pathogens such as *Escherichia coli* and *Salmonella*. They do this by producing substances like **bacteriocins**, which inhibit the growth of harmful bacteria, and by competing for nutrients and space within the gut environment, reducing the chance for pathogens to colonize.

Anti-Inflammatory Effects: Probiotics have anti-inflammatory properties that benefit not only the gut but also the body's systemic inflammatory response. Certain strains, such as **Bifidobacterium breve** and **Lactobacillus reuteri**, have been shown to reduce markers of inflammation, which can benefit conditions like irritable bowel syndrome (IBS), inflammatory bowel disease (IBD), and other chronic inflammatory conditions.

Mental Health Benefits: Recent research has highlighted the gut-brain connection, showing that a healthy gut microbiome contributes to better mental health. Probiotics help regulate the production of serotonin and other neurotransmitters that affect mood and stress response. Strains like **Lactobacillus helveticus** and **Bifidobacterium longum** have been studied for their positive impact on anxiety and depression, suggesting that probiotics may support both mental health and immune function.

Modern Advancements in Probiotic Supplementation

While traditional probiotic foods remain beneficial, modern advancements in probiotics have made it possible to take these benefits a step further by isolating specific strains and delivering them in forms that maximize their effectiveness.

Strain-Specific Probiotics: Modern probiotic supplements contain strains that have been clinically tested for specific benefits, such as improving immunity, aiding digestion, or reducing inflammation. For example, **Lactobacillus rhamnosus GG** is a well-researched strain known for its ability to reduce the duration and severity of gastrointestinal infections, while **Bifidobacterium lactis BB-12** is widely used to support immune function.

Enteric Coating and Delayed-Release Capsules: Probiotics are sensitive to stomach acid, which can destroy many of the beneficial bacteria before they reach the intestines. Enteric-coated capsules and delayed-release technology protect the bacteria as they pass through the stomach, ensuring that more of them survive and reach the intestines intact, where they can have the most impact.

Prebiotics: Prebiotics are fibers that serve as food for probiotics, helping beneficial bacteria to thrive in the gut. Modern supplements often combine probiotics with prebiotics (known as **synbiotics**) to improve the survival and colonization of the probiotics. Foods high in prebiotic fibers, like garlic, onions, and bananas, can also be added to traditional probiotic-rich diets to support a healthy gut environment.

High-Potency and Multi-Strain Formulas: High-potency probiotics with billions of CFUs (colony-forming units) and multiple strains have become popular for providing a broad-spectrum approach to gut health and immunity. Multi-strain formulas offer a diversity of benefits, as different strains target various aspects of digestion, immunity, and overall health.

Shelf-Stable Probiotics: Some probiotic strains are now developed to be shelf-stable, meaning they do not require refrigeration. This makes them more convenient for daily use and travel, ensuring individuals can support their gut health consistently.

Integrating Traditional and Modern Probiotics for Enhanced Health Benefits

Combining traditional probiotic-rich foods with modern probiotic supplements offers a comprehensive approach to digestive and immune health. Here are some practical ways to integrate both:

Daily Probiotic-Rich Foods: Including a serving of yogurt, sauerkraut, kimchi, or kefir in daily meals provides a natural source of beneficial bacteria and adds variety to the diet. These foods offer a range of bacterial strains that can support a balanced gut microbiome.

Targeted Supplementation: For specific health concerns, such as recurring infections, digestive issues, or immune support, adding a high-potency, multi-strain probiotic supplement can enhance the effects of probiotic foods. Choose supplements with clinically studied strains for best results.

Prebiotics for Optimal Gut Health: Combining prebiotic foods like garlic, onions, and oats with probiotic-rich foods or supplements encourages beneficial bacteria to thrive. Prebiotics ensure a healthy gut environment, boosting the effectiveness of probiotics.

probiotic foods and modern probiotic supplements both play valuable roles in supporting digestion and immunity. By harnessing the power of natural probiotics from foods like yogurt, sauerkraut, and kimchi and combining them with the advancements of modern probiotics, it's possible to create a comprehensive approach to gut health. This synergy between ancient practices and modern science provides a pathway to improved digestion, stronger immunity, and better overall health

These 25 natural recipes have been curated to provide relief from inflammation and pain through the power of traditional ingredients like turmeric, ginger, chamomile, and eucalyptus. Whether applied topically or consumed, each recipe uses ingredients known for their anti-inflammatory effects. You'll find a variety of formats, including compresses, oils, and drinks, that can be easily incorporated into a daily wellness routine. Each recipe also includes modern dosage recommendations and optional variations for enhanced absorption and potency.

25 Natural recipes for pain and inflammation

26. Soothing Turmeric & Ginger Compress

Description: A warm compress to reduce inflammation in sore muscles and joints.
Ingredients:
1 tbsp **turmeric powder**
1 tbsp **ginger powder**
1 cup warm water
A clean cloth or gauze
Instructions:
Mix turmeric and ginger powder in warm water.
Soak the cloth in the mixture, wring it out, and place it over the inflamed area for 15-20 minutes.
Variation:
For Enhanced Absorption: Add 1/2 tsp black pepper to the mixture.
Frequency: Use up to twice daily.

---

27. Golden Milk Anti-Inflammatory Drink

Description: A soothing turmeric latte to reduce internal inflammation.
Ingredients:
1 cup almond milk
1/2 tsp **turmeric powder** (or 1/4 tsp liposomal curcumin)
1/4 tsp cinnamon
A pinch of **black pepper**
1 tsp honey
Instructions:
Warm almond milk and whisk in turmeric, cinnamon, black pepper, and honey.
Pour into a mug and enjoy warm.
Variation:
For Extra Relaxation: Add 1/4 tsp ginger powder.
Frequency: Once daily before bed.

28. Chamomile & Lavender Soak

Description: A relaxing bath soak to ease tension and inflammation.
Ingredients:
1/2 cup dried **chamomile flowers**
1/4 cup dried **lavender flowers**
1 cup Epsom salts
Instructions:
Add chamomile, lavender, and Epsom salts to a warm bath.
Soak for 20-30 minutes to relieve pain and reduce inflammation.
Variation:
For Added Pain Relief: Add 5 drops eucalyptus essential oil.
Frequency: Use 1-2 times per week.

29. Ginger Tea for Joint Pain

Description: A warming tea to alleviate joint inflammation.
Ingredients:
1 tsp **fresh ginger**, grated
1 cup boiling water
1 tsp honey
Instructions:
Steep grated ginger in boiling water for 10 minutes.
Strain, add honey, and enjoy warm.
Variation:
For Extra Immune Support: Add 1/4 tsp lemon juice.
Frequency: Up to 3 times daily.

30. Anti-Inflammatory Turmeric Oil

Description: A massage oil for localized pain relief.
Ingredients:
1/4 cup coconut oil
1 tsp **turmeric powder**
5 drops black pepper essential oil
Instructions:
Warm coconut oil and stir in turmeric and black pepper oil.
Massage onto sore areas and let absorb.
Variation:
For Enhanced Potency: Add 5 drops ginger essential oil.
Frequency: Apply as needed.

31. Peppermint & Eucalyptus Headache Balm

Description: A cooling balm to relieve headache-related inflammation.
Ingredients:
2 tbsp coconut oil
5 drops **peppermint essential oil**
5 drops **eucalyptus essential oil**
Instructions:
Mix oils and apply to temples and back of the neck.
Massage gently and breathe deeply.
Variation:
For Stronger Effect: Add 5 drops lavender essential oil.
Frequency: Use as needed.

32. Anti-Inflammatory Turmeric & Honey Paste

Description: A paste for sore or inflamed skin and joints.
Ingredients:
1 tbsp **turmeric powder**
1 tbsp honey
Instructions:
Mix turmeric powder and honey into a paste.
Apply to affected area, leave for 15 minutes, then rinse.
Variation:
For Increased Absorption: Add a pinch of black pepper.
Frequency: Use once daily.

---

33. Chamomile & Ginger Compress

Description: A gentle compress to ease muscle tension and inflammation.
Ingredients:
1 chamomile tea bag
1/2 tsp grated **ginger**
1 cup hot water
Instructions:
Steep chamomile tea bag and ginger in hot water.
Soak a cloth in the mixture, apply to inflamed area for 15 minutes.
Variation:
For Enhanced Pain Relief: Add 1/2 tsp turmeric powder.
Frequency: Up to twice daily.

---

34. Lemon Ginger Elixir

Description: A refreshing drink to combat inflammation and boost immunity.
Ingredients:
1 cup warm water
1/2 lemon, juiced
1/2 tsp **fresh ginger**, grated
1 tsp honey
Instructions:
Combine all ingredients and stir well.
Drink in the morning for best results.
Variation:
With Turmeric: Add 1/4 tsp turmeric powder.
Frequency: Once daily.

---

35. Arnica & Lavender Muscle Rub

Description: A soothing rub for muscle pain and inflammation.
Ingredients:
1/4 cup arnica oil
5 drops **lavender essential oil**
Instructions:
Mix oils and massage onto sore muscles.
Allow it to absorb for deep relief.
Variation:
For Extra Cooling Effect: Add 5 drops peppermint oil.
Frequency: Apply as needed.

36. Chamomile and Mint Bath Soak

Description: A calming bath soak to ease pain and inflammation.
Ingredients:
1/4 cup dried **chamomile flowers**
1/4 cup dried **mint leaves**
1 cup Epsom salts
Instructions:
Add chamomile, mint, and Epsom salts to a warm bath.
Soak for 20-30 minutes to relieve tension and pain.
Variation:
Add Rosemary: Add 1 tbsp dried rosemary for extra relaxation.
Frequency: Use 1-2 times per week.

---

37. Anti-Inflammatory Turmeric Lemonade

Description: A refreshing turmeric-infused lemonade with anti-inflammatory properties.
Ingredients:
1 cup water
1/4 tsp **turmeric powder**
1/2 lemon, juiced
1 tsp honey
Instructions:
Mix turmeric powder, lemon juice, and honey in water.
Stir well and serve over ice.
Variation:
Enhanced Absorption: Add a pinch of black pepper.
Frequency: Once daily.

---

38. Ginger & Honey Compress for Joint Pain

Description: A warm compress that combines ginger and honey for joint pain relief.
Ingredients:
- 1 tsp grated **ginger**
- 1 tbsp honey
- 1 cup warm water

Instructions:
- Mix ginger and honey in warm water.
- Soak a cloth in the mixture and apply to affected joints for 20 minutes.

Variation:
- **Add Turmeric**: Add 1/4 tsp turmeric powder to the mixture.

Frequency: Use as needed.

---

39. Peppermint & Lavender Foot Soak

Description: A soothing foot soak to reduce inflammation and relieve tired, sore feet.
Ingredients:
- 1/4 cup Epsom salts
- 5 drops **peppermint essential oil**
- 5 drops **lavender essential oil**

Instructions:
- Fill a basin with warm water, add Epsom salts, peppermint, and lavender oils.
- Soak feet for 15-20 minutes.

Variation:
- **Extra Relaxation**: Add 1 tbsp dried chamomile flowers.

Frequency: As needed for relief.

40. Cinnamon & Honey Pain Relief Drink

Description: A warm drink to help ease joint pain and inflammation.
Ingredients:
- 1 cup warm water
- 1/2 tsp **cinnamon powder**
- 1 tsp honey

Instructions:
Stir cinnamon and honey into warm water until dissolved.
Drink in the morning for anti-inflammatory benefits.

Variation:
With Ginger: Add 1/4 tsp grated ginger for extra warmth.

Frequency: Once daily.

---

41. Lavender & Chamomile Sleep Balm

Description: A calming balm to promote relaxation and alleviate tension before sleep.
Ingredients:
- 2 tbsp coconut oil
- 5 drops **lavender essential oil**
- 5 drops **chamomile essential oil**

Instructions:
Mix oils and apply to temples, neck, and wrists before bed.

Variation:
For Enhanced Relaxation: Add 5 drops frankincense oil.

Frequency: Use nightly as needed.

---

42. Apple Cider Vinegar & Ginger Drink

Description: A refreshing tonic to reduce inflammation and support digestion.
Ingredients:
- 1 cup water
- 1 tbsp apple cider vinegar
- 1/2 tsp grated **fresh ginger**
- 1 tsp honey

Instructions:
Mix all ingredients in a glass of water and stir well.

Variation:
Add Turmeric: Add 1/4 tsp turmeric powder for extra anti-inflammatory effects.

Frequency: Once daily in the morning.

---

43. Eucalyptus & Peppermint Massage Oil

Description: A cooling massage oil for relief from sore muscles and tension.
Ingredients:
- 1/4 cup almond oil
- 5 drops **eucalyptus essential oil**
- 5 drops **peppermint essential oil**

Instructions:
Combine oils and massage onto affected areas for cooling relief.

Variation:
For Extra Relaxation: Add 5 drops lavender essential oil.

Frequency: Use as needed.

44. Turmeric & Black Pepper Tea

Description: A tea that combines turmeric and black pepper for enhanced anti-inflammatory benefits.
Ingredients:
- 1 cup water
- 1/2 tsp **turmeric powder**
- A pinch of **black pepper**
- 1 tsp honey

Instructions:
Boil water and add turmeric and black pepper.
Remove from heat, add honey, and enjoy.

Variation:
For Extra Warmth: Add 1/4 tsp grated ginger.
Frequency: Up to twice daily.

---

45. Rosemary & Peppermint Bath Salts

Description: Bath salts that provide relaxation and help reduce muscle soreness and inflammation.
Ingredients:
- 1 cup Epsom salts
- 5 drops **rosemary essential oil**
- 5 drops **peppermint essential oil**

Instructions:
Mix oils with Epsom salts and add to a warm bath.
Soak for 20 minutes to relieve pain and reduce inflammation.

Variation:
Add Lavender: Add 5 drops lavender oil for extra relaxation.
Frequency: Use 1-2 times per week.

---

46. Warm Ginger & Turmeric Elixir

Description: A warming elixir to help ease inflammation and provide immune support.
Ingredients:
1 cup warm water
1/2 tsp **turmeric powder**
1/2 tsp **grated ginger**
1 tsp honey

Instructions:
Combine ingredients and stir until mixed.

Variation:
With Lemon: Add 1/2 lemon, juiced, for additional detox benefits.
Frequency: Once daily.

---

47. Chamomile & Aloe Vera Skin Soothing Gel

Description: A cooling gel for inflamed skin or sore muscles.
Ingredients:
2 tbsp **aloe vera gel**
5 drops **chamomile essential oil**

Instructions:
Mix aloe vera gel and chamomile oil.
Apply to irritated or inflamed areas of the skin.

Variation:
Add Lavender: Add 3 drops lavender oil for extra soothing.
Frequency: Apply as needed.

48. Anti-Inflammatory Rosemary & Lavender Compress

Description: A warm compress to reduce pain and inflammation.
Ingredients:
1 tbsp dried **rosemary**
1 tbsp dried **lavender**
1 cup hot water
Instructions:
Steep rosemary and lavender in hot water for 5 minutes.
Soak a cloth in the infusion, wring out excess water, and place over inflamed area for 15 minutes.
Variation:
Add Chamomile: Add 1 tbsp dried chamomile for added calming effects.
Frequency: Use as needed.

49. Turmeric & Ginger Smoothie

Description: A smoothie to help reduce internal inflammation and boost energy.
Ingredients:
1 cup almond milk
1/2 tsp **turmeric powder**
1/4 tsp **ginger powder**
1/2 banana
1 tbsp honey
Instructions:
Blend all ingredients until smooth and creamy.
Variation:
Enhanced Absorption: Add a pinch of black pepper.
Frequency: Once daily.

50. Peppermint & Ginger Ice Pack for Inflammation

Description: A cooling ice pack infused with peppermint and ginger to relieve pain and inflammation.
Ingredients:
1 cup water
5 drops **peppermint essential oil**
1/2 tsp grated **fresh ginger**
Ice cubes
A clean cloth
Instructions:
Mix water, peppermint oil, and grated ginger.
Place ice cubes in the cloth, pour the mixture over them, and apply to the affected area.
Variation:
Add Eucalyptus Oil: Add 5 drops eucalyptus oil for extra cooling.
Frequency: Use as needed for up to 15 minutes.

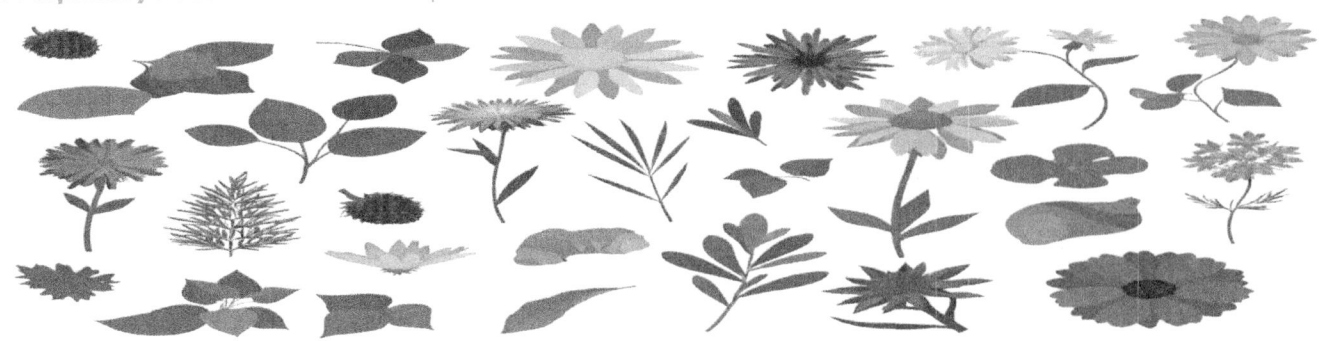

These recipes offer a natural, holistic approach to managing inflammation and pain. From soothing compresses and relaxing soaks to anti-inflammatory drinks, these remedies harness the power of traditional ingredients supported by modern science for enhanced relief._

In our busy world, stress and anxiety are common challenges. These 25 recipes are designed to support mental health and relaxation through the power of nature. Using calming herbs like chamomile, lavender, and valerian, along with soothing essential oils, these infusions, aromatherapy blends, and relaxation drinks offer gentle yet effective ways to promote peace of mind and tranquility. Try incorporating these recipes into your self-care routine for a natural approach to enhancing calm and reducing stress.

25 recipes for mental health and relaxation

51. Chamomile Lavender Sleep Tea
Description: A soothing tea to help calm the mind and prepare for restful sleep.
Ingredients:
1 tsp dried **chamomile flowers**
1 tsp dried **lavender flowers**
1 cup boiling water
Instructions:
Add chamomile and lavender to a teapot or mug, then pour boiling water over.
Steep for 5-7 minutes, strain, and enjoy.
Variation:
Extra Calm: Add 1/4 tsp valerian root for additional sedative effects.
Frequency: Once daily, 30 minutes before bedtime.

52. Relaxing Lemon Balm & Mint Infusion
Description: A calming herbal infusion perfect for reducing stress.
Ingredients:
1 tsp dried **lemon balm**
1 tsp dried **mint leaves**
1 cup hot water
Instructions:
Steep lemon balm and mint in hot water for 5 minutes.
Strain and enjoy warm or over ice.
Variation:
Add Honey: Stir in 1 tsp honey for extra soothing effects.
Frequency: As needed for relaxation.

53. Lavender Aromatherapy Diffuser Blend
Description: A calming blend for relaxation and stress relief.
Ingredients:
3 drops **lavender essential oil**
2 drops **frankincense essential oil**
2 drops **bergamot essential oil**
Instructions:
Add oils to a diffuser with water.
Diffuse for 15-20 minutes to relax the mind.
Variation:
For Uplifting Effect: Add 1 drop orange essential oil.
Frequency: Use as needed.

54. Golden Milk for Relaxation

Description: A warm, soothing drink that promotes relaxation and calms inflammation.
Ingredients:
1 cup almond milk
1/2 tsp **turmeric powder**
1/4 tsp cinnamon
1/4 tsp ginger powder
1 tsp honey
Instructions:
Warm almond milk, then whisk in turmeric, cinnamon, ginger, and honey.
Enjoy warm before bed.
Variation:
For Extra Calm: Add a pinch of nutmeg.
Frequency: Once daily, ideally in the evening.

---

55. Peppermint & Chamomile Foot Soak

Description: A relaxing foot soak to ease tension and promote mental relaxation.
Ingredients:
1/4 cup Epsom salts
5 drops **peppermint essential oil**
5 drops **chamomile essential oil**
Instructions:
Fill a basin with warm water, add Epsom salts and essential oils.
Soak feet for 15-20 minutes.
Variation:
Add Lavender: Add 5 drops lavender essential oil for added relaxation.
Frequency: As needed.

---

56. Honey Chamomile Calming Latte

Description: A gentle, warm chamomile latte that soothes anxiety.
Ingredients:
1 cup oat milk
1 chamomile tea bag
1 tsp honey
Instructions:
Heat oat milk and steep chamomile tea bag for 5 minutes.
Stir in honey and enjoy warm.
Variation:
With Vanilla: Add 1/4 tsp vanilla extract for a richer taste.
Frequency: Once daily.

---

57. Frankincense & Lavender Calm Balm

Description: A calming balm for temples and wrists to promote relaxation.
Ingredients:
2 tbsp coconut oil
5 drops **frankincense essential oil**
5 drops **lavender essential oil**
Instructions:
Mix oils and store in a small container.
Apply to temples and wrists as needed.
Variation:
Add Cedarwood: Add 3 drops cedarwood oil for grounding.
Frequency: Use as needed.

58. Valerian Root Sleep Elixir

Description: A potent drink to ease anxiety and support sleep.
Ingredients:
1/4 tsp dried **valerian root**
1 cup boiling water
1 tsp honey
Instructions:
Steep valerian root in boiling water for 10 minutes.
Strain, add honey, and enjoy 30 minutes before bed.
Variation:
Milder Option: Use 1/8 tsp valerian root if sensitive.
Frequency: Once daily before sleep.

---

59. Mindfulness Rose & Bergamot Spray

Description: A calming mist to use for mindfulness or meditation.
Ingredients:
1/2 cup distilled water
5 drops **rose essential oil**
5 drops **bergamot essential oil**
Instructions:
Combine ingredients in a spray bottle.
Mist in your space or onto your body before meditation.
Variation:
Add Lavender: Add 3 drops lavender oil for extra calm.
Frequency: Use as desired.

---

60. Lemon Balm & Chamomile Calming Tea

Description: A gentle tea to reduce anxiety and enhance mental clarity.
Ingredients:
1 tsp dried **lemon balm**
1 tsp dried **chamomile**
1 cup hot water
Instructions:
Steep herbs in hot water for 5-7 minutes.
Strain and enjoy warm.
Variation:
Add Mint: Add a few fresh mint leaves for a refreshing twist.
Frequency: Up to twice daily.

---

61. Peppermint & Eucalyptus Shower Melt

Description: A calming shower melt for refreshing, anxiety-relieving steam.
Ingredients:
1 cup baking soda
10 drops **peppermint essential oil**
5 drops **eucalyptus essential oil**
Instructions:
Mix ingredients and form small balls.
Place a melt in the shower for a relaxing steam.
Variation:
Add Lavender: Add 5 drops lavender essential oil.
Frequency: Use as desired.

62. Vanilla & Lavender Relaxation Latte

Description: A comforting drink to soothe nerves and enhance relaxation.
Ingredients:
1 cup coconut milk
1/2 tsp **vanilla extract**
1/2 tsp dried **lavender flowers**
1 tsp honey
Instructions:
Heat coconut milk with lavender flowers; strain.
Stir in vanilla and honey.
Variation:
Extra Warmth: Add a pinch of cinnamon.
Frequency: Once daily.

63. Frankincense & Cedarwood Meditation Oil

Description: A grounding oil for use during meditation or deep breathing exercises.
Ingredients:
2 tbsp jojoba oil
5 drops **frankincense essential oil**
3 drops **cedarwood essential oil**
Instructions:
Mix oils in a small bottle.
Apply to wrists, temples, or neck before meditation.
Variation:
Add Lavender: Add 3 drops lavender for additional calm.
Frequency: Use as needed.

64. Ashwagandha Relaxation Smoothie (continued)

Description: A smoothie to help reduce stress and support mood balance.
Ingredients:
1 cup almond milk
1/2 banana
1/2 tsp **ashwagandha powder**
1 tbsp almond butter
1 tsp honey (optional)
Instructions:
Blend all ingredients until smooth.
Serve immediately.
Variation:
Add Vanilla: Add 1/4 tsp vanilla extract for extra flavor.
Frequency: Once daily, ideally in the morning or afternoon.

65. Calming Chamomile & Rose Bath Soak

Description: A relaxing bath soak to ease tension and soothe the mind.
Ingredients:
1/2 cup dried **chamomile flowers**
1/4 cup dried **rose petals**
1 cup Epsom salts
Instructions:
Add chamomile, rose petals, and Epsom salts to a warm bath.
Soak for 20-30 minutes to relax and unwind.
Variation:
Add Lavender: Add 1/4 cup dried lavender for additional calming effects.
Frequency: As needed, up to twice per week.

66. Valerian & Lemon Balm Sleep Tincture

Description: A calming tincture to promote relaxation and support sleep.
Ingredients:
1/2 tsp **valerian root** tincture
1/2 tsp **lemon balm** tincture
1/4 cup water
Instructions:
Mix valerian and lemon balm tinctures with water.
Drink 30 minutes before bedtime.
Variation:
For Milder Effect: Use 1/4 tsp valerian root tincture if sensitive.
Frequency: Once nightly.

---

67. Lavender Vanilla Room Spray

Description: A gentle room spray to create a calm and relaxing atmosphere.
Ingredients:
1 cup distilled water
5 drops **lavender essential oil**
3 drops **vanilla essential oil**
Instructions:
Combine all ingredients in a spray bottle and shake well.
Mist lightly around your room or space.
Variation:
Add Rose: Add 3 drops rose essential oil for added calm.
Frequency: Use as needed.

---

68. Chamomile & Peppermint Pillow Spray

Description: A relaxing pillow spray to help prepare for restful sleep.
Ingredients:
1/2 cup distilled water
5 drops **chamomile essential oil**
3 drops **peppermint essential oil**
Instructions:
Combine ingredients in a spray bottle.
Lightly mist your pillow before bedtime.
Variation:
Add Lavender: Add 2 drops lavender essential oil for added relaxation.
Frequency: Nightly as desired.

---

69. Lavender Honey Calming Milk

Description: A warm, comforting drink with lavender and honey for mental relaxation.
Ingredients:
1 cup warm milk (any variety)
1/2 tsp dried **lavender flowers**
1 tsp honey
Instructions:
Heat milk and add lavender flowers. Let steep for 5 minutes, then strain.
Stir in honey and enjoy warm.
Variation:
With Vanilla: Add 1/4 tsp vanilla extract for added flavor.
Frequency: Once daily, preferably in the evening.

70. Peppermint & Rosemary Clarity Spray

Description: A refreshing spray to boost mental clarity and calm anxiety.
Ingredients:
1/2 cup distilled water
5 drops **peppermint essential oil**
3 drops **rosemary essential oil**
Instructions:
Combine ingredients in a spray bottle and shake well.
Mist lightly around your workspace for focus and calm.
Variation:
Add Lemon: Add 2 drops lemon essential oil for a bright, uplifting scent.
Frequency: As needed for focus and clarity.

---

71. Lemon Balm & Ginger Calming Elixir

Description: A warm elixir to reduce anxiety and calm the mind.
Ingredients:
1 tsp dried **lemon balm**
1/2 tsp **fresh ginger**, grated
1 cup hot water
1 tsp honey
Instructions:
Steep lemon balm and ginger in hot water for 5 minutes.
Strain, add honey, and enjoy warm.
Variation:
Add Cinnamon: Add a pinch of cinnamon for extra warmth.
Frequency: Up to twice daily.

---

72. Calming Rose & Lavender Tea

Description: A floral tea to calm the mind and soothe the senses.
Ingredients:
1 tsp dried **rose petals**
1/2 tsp dried **lavender flowers**
1 cup boiling water
Instructions:
Steep rose petals and lavender in boiling water for 5 minutes.
Strain and enjoy warm.
Variation:
Add Chamomile: Add 1/2 tsp dried chamomile for added relaxation.
Frequency: As desired.

73. Lavender & Eucalyptus Stress-Relief Roll-On

Description: A portable roll-on for quick stress relief.
Ingredients:
10 ml roller bottle
5 drops **lavender essential oil**
3 drops **eucalyptus essential oil**
Carrier oil (such as almond oil)
Instructions:
Add essential oils to roller bottle, fill with carrier oil, and shake.
Roll onto wrists and temples for instant calm.
Variation:
Add Bergamot: Add 2 drops bergamot for extra soothing.
Frequency: Use as needed.

---

74. Passionflower & Chamomile Relaxation Tea

Description: A gentle tea to reduce anxiety and promote relaxation.
Ingredients:
1/2 tsp dried **passionflower**
1/2 tsp dried **chamomile**
1 cup hot water
Instructions:
Steep passionflower and chamomile in hot water for 5-7 minutes.
Strain and enjoy warm.
Variation:
Add Lemon Balm: Add 1/4 tsp dried lemon balm for extra calming effects.
Frequency: Once daily, in the evening.

---

75. 2Calming Holy Basil (Tulsi) Tea

Description: A traditional herbal tea to reduce stress and support mental balance.
Ingredients:
1 tsp dried **holy basil (tulsi) leaves**
1 cup hot water
Instructions:
Steep holy basil leaves in hot water for 5-7 minutes.
Strain and enjoy warm.
Variation:
Add Mint: Add a few fresh mint leaves for added freshness.
Frequency: Up to twice daily.

These recipes provide natural ways to enhance mental relaxation and support overall well-being, using gentle yet effective ingredients known for their calming properties. From comforting teas to soothing sprays and balms, these recipes can be easily integrated into a daily routine to help reduce stress and promote peace of mind.

Chapter 5

Natural Remedies and Skin Care

For Skin Care: Traditional Treatments with Aloe Vera, Tea Tree, Coconut Oil, and Other Natural Remedies

Our skin is constantly exposed to environmental stressors, and caring for it with natural, gentle remedies is a time-honored approach to maintaining health and radiance. Traditional skincare treatments using ingredients like **aloe vera, tea tree oil**, and **coconut oil** have been cherished for their effectiveness in soothing, nourishing, and healing the skin. These natural remedies contain potent compounds that support skin health, fight bacteria, reduce inflammation, and provide essential hydration without harsh chemicals. Here's an overview of these natural skincare wonders and how they work:

Aloe Vera: The Healing Plant

Aloe vera has been used for centuries to treat a variety of skin ailments. Known for its cooling and moisturizing properties, aloe vera is rich in **polysaccharides, vitamins, and antioxidants** that support skin healing. Its benefits include:

Soothing Burns and Sunburns: Aloe vera's cooling effect helps reduce redness and inflammation associated with sunburns. Applying aloe gel directly to burned skin can speed up healing and minimize discomfort.

Hydrating and Calming Sensitive Skin: Aloe vera provides lightweight hydration without clogging pores, making it ideal for sensitive or acne-prone skin. The gel can be applied directly to the face to calm irritation and redness.

Reducing Acne Scarring: Aloe's ability to stimulate collagen production helps reduce the appearance of scars and blemishes over time.

How to Use Aloe Vera: Use fresh aloe vera gel directly from the plant or a pure, additive-free aloe vera gel for best results. Apply it directly to cleansed skin as a daily moisturizer, leave-on mask, or soothing spot treatment.

Tea Tree Oil: Nature's Antimicrobial Powerhouse

Tea tree oil, extracted from the leaves of the Melaleuca alternifolia tree, has strong antibacterial and anti-inflammatory properties. It has been traditionally used to combat acne, reduce skin infections, and heal cuts and scrapes. The main benefits of tea tree oil include:

Treating Acne and Blemishes: Tea tree oil is highly effective in reducing acne due to its antimicrobial properties. It helps target *Propionibacterium acnes*, the bacteria responsible for acne, without over-drying the skin.

Soothing Insect Bites and Minor Cuts: The anti-inflammatory effect of tea tree oil can reduce redness and swelling from insect bites, minor cuts, and scrapes.

Controlling Excess Oil: Tea tree oil helps regulate sebum production, making it suitable for oily and combination skin types.

How to Use Tea Tree Oil: Dilute tea tree oil with a carrier oil (such as coconut or jojoba oil) before applying it to the skin to prevent irritation. It can be used as a spot treatment for acne or added to a face wash for gentle cleansing.

Coconut Oil: The Deep Moisturizer

Coconut oil has been a staple in traditional skincare for centuries, especially in tropical regions. Rich in **fatty acids and antioxidants**, it deeply hydrates, nourishes, and protects the skin. Key benefits of coconut oil include:

Moisturizing Dry Skin: Coconut oil penetrates deep into the skin, providing long-lasting hydration for dry and flaky skin.

Antibacterial and Anti-Fungal Properties: Coconut oil contains lauric acid, which has antimicrobial properties that can help prevent infections and skin irritation.

Reducing the Appearance of Wrinkles: The antioxidants in coconut oil help protect the skin from free radicals, reducing signs of aging such as fine lines and wrinkles.

How to Use Coconut Oil: Apply a small amount of coconut oil as a natural moisturizer, especially on dry areas like elbows, knees, and heels. Avoid using it on acne-prone areas, as it can be comedogenic for some skin types.

Other Natural Skin Remedies

In addition to aloe vera, tea tree, and coconut oil, several other traditional remedies offer remarkable skin benefits:

Honey: Known for its antibacterial and humectant properties, honey is excellent for soothing, moisturizing, and healing the skin. Manuka honey, in particular, has potent healing abilities and can be used as a spot treatment for acne or a face mask for hydration.

Jojoba Oil: This lightweight oil mimics the skin's natural sebum, making it suitable for all skin types, including oily and acne-prone skin. It's non-comedogenic, deeply hydrating, and can help balance oil production.

Witch Hazel: Derived from the bark and leaves of the witch hazel shrub, this natural astringent is excellent for reducing inflammation, tightening pores, and controlling excess oil. It's often used as a toner for oily and combination skin.

Shea Butter: Known for its high concentration of vitamins and fatty acids, shea butter provides deep hydration and is especially beneficial for very dry, cracked skin. It also has anti-inflammatory properties, making it suitable for soothing eczema and dermatitis.

Rose Water: Rose water is a gentle toner with anti-inflammatory and hydrating properties. It's ideal for sensitive or irritated skin, helping to soothe redness and refresh the complexion.

How to Create a Simple Natural Skincare Routine

Using these natural remedies, you can create a gentle skincare routine that supports skin health without the use of harsh chemicals. Here's a basic guide to incorporating these ingredients into a daily skincare regimen:

Cleanse: Use a gentle cleanser suitable for your skin type. For acne-prone or oily skin, consider adding a few drops of tea tree oil to your face wash.

Tone: Use witch hazel or rose water as a toner to balance the skin's pH and tighten pores.

Moisturize: Apply aloe vera gel as a lightweight moisturizer for oily or sensitive skin, or use jojoba or coconut oil for deeper hydration on dry skin.

Spot Treatment: For acne, use a diluted tea tree oil on blemishes or a dab of Manuka honey for targeted healing.

Weekly Mask: Apply a honey and aloe vera mask once a week to soothe and hydrate the skin.

Traditional skincare ingredients like aloe vera, tea tree, and coconut oil have stood the test of time for their effectiveness and safety. By using these natural remedies in combination with a simple, consistent routine, you can nurture and protect your skin, maintaining a healthy, radiant complexion without unnecessary additives. Whether you're looking to soothe irritation, hydrate dry skin, or control acne, these natural ingredients offer a reliable foundation for gentle, effective skincare.

Modern Dermatology and Enhancements: How Modern Medicine Has Refined the Use of These Remedies for Specific Skin Issues like Acne, Wrinkles, and Irritations

Modern dermatology has leveraged scientific advancements to refine and enhance the traditional use of natural remedies such as aloe vera, tea tree oil, and coconut oil. By applying rigorous research and controlled studies, dermatologists have optimized these natural treatments to address specific skin issues such as acne, wrinkles, and irritations with more precision and effectiveness. Here's a closer look at how modern medicine has adapted these traditional ingredients to provide targeted skincare solutions.

Aloe Vera for Acne and Skin Irritations

Aloe vera, long known for its soothing properties, has become a staple in modern dermatology for treating acne and irritation. Scientific studies have revealed that **aloe vera's compounds—polysaccharides, antioxidants, and enzymes**—not only reduce inflammation but also enhance wound healing. These insights have allowed dermatologists to use aloe vera in more focused ways to improve skin health:

Acne Treatment: Modern dermatology combines aloe vera with proven acne-fighting ingredients like **salicylic acid** and **benzoyl peroxide** to reduce inflammation while promoting skin healing. Aloe vera's gentle, hydrating nature counteracts the dryness often caused by harsher acne treatments, making it ideal for sensitive skin.

Soothing Eczema and Psoriasis: Thanks to its hydrating and anti-inflammatory properties, aloe vera is commonly included in creams and gels for eczema and psoriasis. Clinical research has shown that aloe can alleviate itchiness and reduce redness, providing relief for those with chronic skin conditions.

Burn and Wound Healing: Aloe vera gels are now formulated with improved delivery systems that allow its healing compounds to penetrate deeper into the skin. These formulations are used in hospitals and clinics for burn treatment and to speed up wound recovery.

Example of Modern Aloe Vera Product: Medical-grade aloe vera gels, often enhanced with liposomal technology, deliver deeper hydration and faster relief from irritation than traditional aloe products.

Tea Tree Oil for Acne and Oily Skin

Tea tree oil's natural antibacterial and anti-inflammatory properties have made it a popular choice for treating acne. Modern dermatology has refined tea tree oil's use to maximize its effectiveness against acne-causing bacteria while minimizing the risk of skin irritation:

Spot Treatment for Acne: Dermatologists recommend using tea tree oil in a diluted form, often as a spot treatment, to target active breakouts. Studies have shown that **5% tea tree oil formulations** are effective against mild to moderate acne and comparable in effectiveness to benzoyl peroxide, but with fewer side effects.

Balancing Oil Production: Formulations that blend tea tree oil with lightweight carrier oils (like jojoba oil) or non-comedogenic bases provide acne-prone skin with hydration without clogging pores. This approach regulates oil production, reducing both acne breakouts and skin shine.

Reducing Inflammation and Post-Acne Scars: By combining tea tree oil with ingredients like **niacinamide** and **azelaic acid**, modern formulations reduce redness and prevent post-inflammatory hyperpigmentation, helping to fade acne scars over time.

Example of Modern Tea Tree Product: Tea tree oil-based cleansers, gels, and serums are carefully formulated with balanced concentrations to avoid irritation while delivering powerful antibacterial benefits.

Coconut Oil for Wrinkles and Dry Skin

Coconut oil has been known for its moisturizing and anti-aging properties, but modern dermatology has improved its application by understanding its fatty acid profile and potential for skin repair. While coconut oil is particularly beneficial for dry and mature skin, it has been optimized to be safer for use on the face through formulation advances:

Anti-Aging Benefits: Coconut oil is rich in **lauric acid** and **antioxidants**, which help protect the skin from oxidative damage, a major contributor to wrinkles. Dermatologists now combine coconut oil with **vitamin E** and other antioxidants to create formulations that address fine lines and improve skin elasticity.

Deep Moisture for Dry Skin: Coconut oil-based moisturizers and creams are refined to ensure penetration into the skin's deeper layers, providing lasting hydration. This approach prevents water loss and repairs the skin's barrier, making it ideal for treating chronic dry skin and conditions like eczema.

Safer Use for Sensitive or Acne-Prone Skin: While coconut oil can be comedogenic for some skin types, modern formulations blend it with non-comedogenic oils or add ingredients like **squalane** and **hyaluronic acid** to maintain moisture without clogging pores. This makes it safer for individuals with sensitive or acne-prone skin.

Example of Modern Coconut Oil Product: Lightweight coconut oil serums with added hyaluronic acid or water-based emulsions offer deep hydration without heaviness, benefiting both dry and sensitive skin.

Other Natural Ingredients Enhanced by Modern Dermatology

Modern dermatology has also embraced and optimized additional natural ingredients, using scientific research to improve their efficacy for specific skin concerns:

Witch Hazel for Oil Control and Reducing Pores: Traditionally known as an astringent, witch hazel has been refined to reduce irritation while effectively controlling oil production and tightening pores. Formulations that combine witch hazel with **soothing agents like aloe vera** or **panthenol** are especially beneficial for oily and combination skin.

Shea Butter for Wrinkles and Skin Repair: Shea butter is a rich source of fatty acids and antioxidants, providing intense moisture and repair for damaged skin. Dermatologists now use purified forms of shea butter in anti-aging creams and add active ingredients like **peptides** to enhance collagen production, making it more effective for mature skin.

Rosehip Oil for Anti-Aging and Scar Reduction: Rich in **vitamin A** and **essential fatty acids**, rosehip oil is widely used in modern dermatology to treat scars, pigmentation, and fine lines. Formulations that blend rosehip oil with **retinoids** or **vitamin C** offer a gentle yet potent option for skin rejuvenation and evening skin tone.

Combining Traditional Remedies with Advanced Dermatological Ingredients

The integration of traditional remedies with modern active ingredients and delivery systems has given dermatologists new tools to tackle complex skin issues. Here are some examples of how these combinations can work to enhance skin health:

Aloe Vera and Hyaluronic Acid for Sensitive, Dehydrated Skin: The soothing properties of aloe vera, combined with hyaluronic acid, provide lightweight hydration without irritation, ideal for those with sensitive skin or rosacea. This combination supports both moisture retention and inflammation reduction.

Tea Tree Oil and Salicylic Acid for Acne Control: This pairing combines tea tree oil's antibacterial properties with salicylic acid's exfoliating effects, creating a powerful yet gentle treatment for acne-prone skin. It targets bacteria, unclogs pores, and reduces redness for a clearer complexion.

Coconut Oil and Peptides for Anti-Aging: Coconut oil's moisturizing benefits are enhanced by peptides, which stimulate collagen production to reduce fine lines. This combination works well for mature or dry skin, providing both hydration and anti-aging support.

Shea Butter and Retinol for Nightly Skin Repair: Shea butter deeply nourishes the skin while retinol encourages cell turnover, helping to repair damage and reduce signs of aging. Together, they create a balanced, nourishing formula that smooths wrinkles and improves skin texture.

By refining and enhancing natural ingredients with the support of scientific research, modern dermatology has expanded the possibilities for skin care using traditional remedies. Today's formulations harness the full potential of aloe vera, tea tree oil, coconut oil, and other natural ingredients to address specific skin concerns like acne, wrinkles, and irritations more effectively. With the precise application of these remedies, dermatologists offer a balanced approach to skin health that honors the wisdom of nature while maximizing efficacy through modern innovations.

Combined Skincare Routine: Practical Tips for Integrating Traditional Remedies and Modern Products

Creating a skincare routine that combines traditional remedies and modern products allows you to enjoy the best of both worlds. Traditional ingredients like aloe vera, tea tree oil, and coconut oil provide gentle, natural benefits, while modern products introduce scientifically backed active ingredients and advanced formulations. This balanced approach can help address a variety of skin needs, from hydration and anti-aging to acne and soothing inflammation. Here's a practical guide to integrating traditional remedies and modern skincare products into a cohesive, effective routine:

Morning Routine
Cleanse Gently with Natural and Modern Cleansers
   Traditional: Start with a gentle wash using natural ingredients like honey, which has antibacterial properties and is suitable for all skin types, especially those prone to acne or sensitivity. Simply massage a small amount of honey onto damp skin, then rinse with lukewarm water.
   Modern: If you prefer a traditional cleanser, look for one with gentle exfoliating properties or ingredients like **salicylic acid** (for oily/acne-prone skin) or **hyaluronic acid** (for dry skin). Combining this with natural cleansing can keep your skin clear without stripping away moisture.

Tone with Witch Hazel and Modern Toners
   Traditional: Witch hazel has natural astringent properties, which can help to refine pores and control oil without harsh chemicals. Use a few drops on a cotton pad and apply to the T-zone or any area where oiliness is common.
   Modern: Follow with a modern toner containing ingredients like **niacinamide** or **vitamin C** to brighten the skin and provide antioxidant protection. Niacinamide can be paired with witch hazel to reduce oil and help maintain even skin tone.

Apply a Lightweight Moisturizer or Gel with Aloe Vera
>**Traditional**: Aloe vera gel is lightweight, hydrating, and soothing, making it ideal for daytime use, especially in warm climates. Apply a thin layer to moisturize and prep the skin for further products.
>
>**Modern**: Look for a moisturizer with ingredients like **hyaluronic acid** or **ceramides** for extra hydration and skin barrier support. These can be layered over aloe vera for added moisture without feeling heavy.

Protect with Sunscreen
>**Modern**: Sunscreen is one of the most critical steps in any skincare routine. Choose a broad-spectrum SPF of at least 30 to protect against UV damage, which can exacerbate skin issues like hyperpigmentation, wrinkles, and dryness. Look for sunscreens with **zinc oxide** or **titanium dioxide** for physical protection that's less likely to irritate sensitive skin.
>
>**Tip**: If using natural oils, such as coconut oil for hydration, apply these at night rather than under sunscreen, as oils can decrease sunscreen effectiveness.

Evening Routine

Double Cleanse to Remove Impurities
>**Traditional**: Start with an oil cleanse using coconut or jojoba oil to dissolve makeup and impurities. Massage a small amount onto dry skin, then wipe away with a warm, damp cloth.
>
>**Modern**: Follow with a gentle, pH-balanced cleanser to remove any remaining residue and prepare the skin for treatments. This step ensures a deep cleanse without stripping the skin of essential moisture.

Exfoliate with Natural and Modern Exfoliants
>**Traditional**: Use a mild exfoliating treatment, such as a mixture of ground oatmeal and honey, once or twice a week. Oatmeal is gentle and helps slough away dead skin while soothing inflammation.
>
>**Modern**: Alternatively, incorporate an exfoliating serum containing **AHAs** (alpha hydroxy acids) like glycolic or lactic acid once or twice a week. These acids provide deeper exfoliation to smooth texture and brighten skin tone, complementing the gentle effect of natural exfoliants.

Target Treatment with Tea Tree Oil and Serums
>**Traditional**: For acne-prone skin, apply diluted tea tree oil as a spot treatment on blemishes. It's naturally antibacterial and helps reduce inflammation without harsh chemicals.
>
>**Modern**: Layer on a serum containing **retinoids** or **vitamin C** to address issues like fine lines, dark spots, or uneven texture. Retinoids stimulate cell turnover and collagen production, while vitamin C brightens and protects against environmental stressors.

Moisturize with Coconut Oil and Night Creams
>**Traditional**: Apply a small amount of coconut oil to dry areas (like cheeks and forehead) to deeply hydrate and lock in moisture overnight. Coconut oil provides a natural barrier that nourishes and softens the skin.

Modern: Follow with a night cream that includes **peptides** or **ceramides** for additional skin barrier repair and anti-aging support. The combination of coconut oil and peptides helps smooth and hydrate skin without clogging pores.

Weekly Masking with Shea Butter and Hydrating Masks

Traditional: Once a week, apply a shea butter mask for deep hydration and soothing. Shea butter is rich in vitamins and antioxidants that support the skin's elasticity and hydration.

Modern: Use a modern hydrating or detox mask, such as one containing **hyaluronic acid** or **charcoal**, on alternate weeks. Hydrating masks restore moisture, while detox masks draw out impurities, making them a perfect complement to shea butter's nourishing effects.

General Tips for Combining Traditional and Modern Skincare

Layer Mindfully: Always start with the lightest textures (such as gels and serums) and finish with thicker, occlusive products like oils or shea butter. This approach ensures that active ingredients penetrate effectively and that moisture is locked in for optimal hydration.

Patch Test New Combinations: When integrating modern actives like retinoids or vitamin C with traditional remedies, patch test on a small area to check for any potential irritation. While many natural remedies are gentle, certain combinations can be too potent for sensitive skin types.

Alternate Treatments to Avoid Over-Exfoliation: To prevent skin irritation, avoid layering multiple active ingredients, such as AHAs, retinoids, or tea tree oil, in a single routine. Instead, alternate these treatments on different nights to allow your skin time to recover and benefit from each product.

Balance Hydration and Treatment: Modern active ingredients, like retinoids or salicylic acid, can be drying, especially when first introduced. Balance these treatments with hydrating traditional ingredients like aloe vera and coconut oil to maintain moisture and soothe any irritation.

Customize for Skin Type and Concerns: For oily or acne-prone skin, focus on lighter layers, like aloe vera gel, witch hazel, and lightweight serums, to reduce shine and breakouts. For dry or mature skin, incorporate richer oils like coconut oil and shea butter along with peptide or hyaluronic acid-rich serums for added nourishment.

By thoughtfully combining traditional remedies and modern skincare products, you can create a comprehensive routine that addresses multiple skin concerns while supporting long-term skin health. This balanced approach not only leverages the power of nature but also benefits from the science-backed advancements in dermatology, ensuring that your skin receives gentle yet effective care.

Here is a curated collection of 25 natural skincare recipes designed to nourish, soothe, and rejuvenate the skin using the gentle power of ingredients like aloe vera, honey, tea tree oil, and various essential oils. These recipes provide effective solutions for different skincare needs—from hydrating masks and exfoliating scrubs to calming oils and spot treatments. Each recipe includes easy-to-follow instructions, variations to tailor the treatments to specific skin types, and optimal application methods for achieving radiant, healthy skin.

25 skin care recipes

76. **1. Aloe Vera & Honey Hydrating Face Mask**

Description: A hydrating mask that soothes and moisturizes skin.
Ingredients:
   2 tbsp fresh **aloe vera gel**
   1 tbsp **honey**
Instructions:
   Mix aloe vera gel and honey until smooth.
   Apply an even layer to clean skin and leave on for 15-20 minutes.
   Rinse with warm water and pat dry.
Variation:
   Add Vitamin E: Add 1 capsule of vitamin E for extra nourishment.
Frequency: Use 1-2 times per week.

---

77. **2. Tea Tree Oil Spot Treatment for Acne**

Description: A powerful spot treatment for acne-prone skin.
Ingredients:
   1 drop **tea tree essential oil**
   1 tsp **aloe vera gel** or **jojoba oil**
Instructions:
   Mix tea tree oil with aloe vera gel or jojoba oil.
   Apply a small amount to blemishes using a cotton swab.
   Leave on overnight; rinse in the morning.
Variation:
   Diluted Option: Use 2 drops tea tree oil with 2 tsp aloe vera for sensitive skin.
Frequency: As needed for spot treatment.

---

78. **3. Honey & Sugar Exfoliating Face Scrub**

Description: A gentle scrub to smooth and brighten the skin.
Ingredients:
   1 tbsp **honey**
   1 tbsp **sugar**
Instructions:
   Combine honey and sugar.
   Gently massage onto damp skin in circular motions.
   Rinse with warm water and follow with moisturizer.
Variation:
   Add Lemon: Add 1/2 tsp lemon juice for a brightening effect.
Frequency: Once a week.

79. 4. Oatmeal & Aloe Calming Mask for Sensitive Skin

Description: A soothing mask to reduce redness and irritation.
Ingredients:
- 1 tbsp **oatmeal**, finely ground
- 1 tbsp **aloe vera gel**

Instructions:
- Mix ground oatmeal and aloe vera until you get a paste.
- Apply to the face and leave on for 15 minutes.
- Rinse with cool water.

Variation:
- **Add Chamomile**: Add 1 tsp chamomile tea for extra calming.

Frequency: As needed.

---

80. 5. Coconut Oil & Honey Deep Moisturizing Mask

Description: A deeply hydrating mask for dry or mature skin.
Ingredients:
- 1 tbsp **coconut oil**
- 1 tbsp **honey**

Instructions:
- Mix coconut oil and honey.
- Apply to the face, leave on for 15-20 minutes.
- Rinse with warm water.

Variation:
- **Add Avocado**: Mash 1/4 avocado for added nutrients.

Frequency: Once a week.

---

81. 6. Green Tea & Honey Antioxidant Mask

Description: An antioxidant-rich mask to protect and rejuvenate.
Ingredients:
- 1 tbsp brewed, cooled **green tea**
- 1 tbsp **honey**

Instructions:
- Mix green tea and honey.
- Apply to the face and leave on for 15 minutes.
- Rinse with cool water.

Variation:
- **Add Aloe**: Add 1 tsp aloe vera gel for hydration.

Frequency: 1-2 times per week.

---

82. 7. Avocado & Honey Nourishing Mask

Description: A nutrient-rich mask for dry or mature skin.
Ingredients:
- 1/4 ripe **avocado**, mashed
- 1 tbsp **honey**

Instructions:
- Mix mashed avocado with honey.
- Apply to the face and leave on for 20 minutes.
- Rinse with warm water.

Variation:
- **Add Coconut Oil**: Add 1 tsp coconut oil for deeper hydration.

Frequency: Weekly.

83.   8. Baking Soda & Honey Clarifying Scrub

Description: A gentle scrub to cleanse and exfoliate.
Ingredients:
- 1 tbsp **baking soda**
- 1 tbsp **honey**

Instructions:
- Combine baking soda and honey to form a paste.
- Gently massage onto skin and rinse.

Variation:
- **Add Aloe Vera**: Add 1 tsp aloe vera for a soothing effect.

Frequency: Once a week.

---

84.   9. Yogurt & Honey Brightening Face Mask

Description: A mask to even tone and gently exfoliate.
Ingredients:
- 1 tbsp plain **yogurt**
- 1 tsp **honey**

Instructions:
- Mix yogurt and honey.
- Apply to the face, leave on for 10-15 minutes.
- Rinse with cool water.

Variation:
- **Add Turmeric**: Add a pinch of turmeric for an extra glow.

Frequency: Once weekly.

---

85.   10. Cucumber & Aloe Cooling Mask

Description: A cooling mask to refresh and hydrate.
Ingredients:
- 1 tbsp **aloe vera gel**
- 1 tbsp grated **cucumber**

Instructions:
- Mix aloe vera and cucumber.
- Apply to the face and leave on for 15 minutes.
- Rinse with cool water.

Variation:
- **Add Mint**: Add a few crushed mint leaves for extra freshness.

Frequency: Use as needed.

---

86.   11. Turmeric & Honey Anti-Inflammatory Mask

Description: A mask to reduce inflammation and brighten skin.
Ingredients:
- 1/2 tsp **turmeric powder**
- 1 tbsp **honey**

Instructions:
- Mix turmeric with honey.
- Apply to the face and leave on for 10 minutes.
- Rinse thoroughly to avoid staining.

Variation:
- **Add Yogurt**: Add 1 tbsp yogurt for extra soothing.

Frequency: Once a week.

87. 12. Olive Oil & Sugar Exfoliating Body Scrub

Description: A hydrating scrub to smooth and soften the skin.
Ingredients:
- 1 tbsp **olive oil**
- 1 tbsp **sugar**

Instructions:
- Mix olive oil and sugar.
- Gently scrub onto damp skin in circular motions, focusing on dry areas.
- Rinse with warm water and pat dry.

Variation:
- **Add Honey**: Add 1 tsp honey for added hydration.

Frequency: Weekly.

---

88. 13. Coconut & Lavender Calming Night Oil

Description: A nourishing oil for dry or irritated skin.
Ingredients:
- 1 tbsp **coconut oil**
- 3 drops **lavender essential oil**

Instructions:
- Mix oils together.
- Apply a small amount to face or dry areas before bedtime.

Variation:
- **Add Rosehip Oil**: Add 1 tsp rosehip oil for extra anti-aging benefits.

Frequency: Nightly as needed.

---

89. 14. Honey & Lemon Brightening Mask

Description: A brightening mask for dull skin.
Ingredients:
- 1 tbsp **honey**
- 1/2 tsp **lemon juice**

Instructions:
- Mix honey and lemon juice.
- Apply to the face, leave for 10 minutes, then rinse.

Variation:
- **Add Yogurt**: Add 1 tbsp yogurt for gentle exfoliation.

Frequency: Use once a week.

---

90. 15. Tea Tree & Aloe Oil-Control Mask (continued)

Instructions:
- Mix aloe vera gel with tea tree oil.
- Apply to clean skin, focusing on oily areas.
- Leave on for 15 minutes, then rinse with cool water.

Variation:
- **Add Clay**: Add 1 tsp bentonite clay for a deeper cleanse.

Frequency: 1-2 times per week as needed.

91.   16. Banana & Honey Hydrating Mask

Description: A nourishing mask for softening and hydrating dry skin.
Ingredients:
- 1/2 ripe **banana**, mashed
- 1 tbsp **honey**

Instructions:
- Combine mashed banana and honey until smooth.
- Apply to the face, leave for 15-20 minutes, then rinse with warm water.

Variation:
- **Add Yogurt**: Add 1 tbsp yogurt for extra moisturizing.

Frequency: Weekly.

---

92.   17. Rose Water & Aloe Vera Toner

Description: A gentle toner to refresh and soothe the skin.
Ingredients:
- 1/4 cup **rose water**
- 2 tbsp **aloe vera gel**

Instructions:
- Mix rose water and aloe vera in a spray bottle.
- Spritz onto face after cleansing or use with a cotton pad.

Variation:
- **Add Witch Hazel**: Add 1 tbsp witch hazel for oily skin.

Frequency: Use daily.

---

93.   18. Coconut & Coffee Body Scrub

Description: An invigorating body scrub to exfoliate and improve circulation.
Ingredients:
- 2 tbsp **coconut oil**
- 1 tbsp ground **coffee**

Instructions:
- Mix coconut oil and coffee grounds.
- Massage onto damp skin in circular motions, then rinse.

Variation:
- **Add Sugar**: Add 1 tbsp sugar for added exfoliation.

Frequency: Weekly.

---

94.   19. Honey & Cinnamon Acne Mask

Description: A mask to target acne and reduce bacteria.
Ingredients:
- 1 tbsp **honey**
- 1/2 tsp **cinnamon powder**

Instructions:
- Mix honey and cinnamon.
- Apply to acne-prone areas and leave for 10-15 minutes, then rinse.

Variation:
- **Add Tea Tree Oil**: Add 1 drop tea tree oil for extra antibacterial power.

Frequency: 1-2 times per week.

95.   20. Aloe & Cucumber Hydrating Gel

Description: A cooling gel to hydrate and calm the skin.
Ingredients:
- 1/4 cup **aloe vera gel**
- 1 tbsp grated **cucumber**

Instructions:
- Mix aloe vera gel and cucumber.
- Apply a thin layer to the face and leave on; rinse or let it absorb.

Variation:
- **Add Mint**: Add 1 drop peppermint oil for a cooling effect.

Frequency: As needed.

---

96.   21. Shea Butter & Vitamin E Night Cream

Description: A rich cream to deeply nourish and repair skin overnight.
Ingredients:
- 2 tbsp **shea butter**
- 1 tsp **coconut oil**
- 1 capsule of **vitamin E oil**

Instructions:
- Melt shea butter and coconut oil, then mix in vitamin E.
- Apply a small amount to face before bed.

Variation:
- **Add Lavender**: Add 2 drops lavender essential oil for relaxation.

Frequency: Nightly.

---

97.   22. Honey & Oatmeal Gentle Exfoliating Mask

Description: A gentle exfoliating mask for sensitive skin.
Ingredients:
- 1 tbsp **oatmeal**, finely ground
- 1 tbsp **honey**

Instructions:
- Mix ground oatmeal with honey to form a paste.
- Apply to the face, leave for 15 minutes, then rinse with warm water.

Variation:
- **Add Yogurt**: Add 1 tbsp yogurt for additional softness.

Frequency: 1-2 times per week.

---

98.   23. Jojoba & Tea Tree Oil Serum for Acne

Description: A lightweight serum to balance and control acne.
Ingredients:
- 1 tbsp **jojoba oil**
- 2 drops **tea tree oil**

Instructions:
- Mix jojoba oil and tea tree oil.
- Massage a small amount into skin, focusing on oily areas.

Variation:
- **Add Lavender Oil**: Add 1 drop lavender oil for extra calming.

Frequency: Daily or as needed.

99.   24. Honey & Rose Petal Mask for Radiance

Description: A nourishing mask to add radiance to dull skin.
Ingredients:
- 1 tbsp **honey**
- 1 tbsp crushed **rose petals** (or rose water)

Instructions:
- Combine honey and rose petals.
- Apply to the face, leave on for 15 minutes, then rinse.

Variation:
- **Add Yogurt**: Add 1 tbsp yogurt for extra moisture.

Frequency: Weekly.

---

100.   25. Avocado & Olive Oil Hand Cream

Description: A rich hand cream to soften and nourish dry hands.
Ingredients:
- 1/2 ripe **avocado**, mashed
- 1 tbsp **olive oil**

Instructions:
- Mix avocado and olive oil until smooth.
- Apply to hands, leave on for 15-20 minutes, then rinse.

Variation:
- **Add Honey**: Add 1 tsp honey for added hydration.

Frequency: Weekly or as needed.

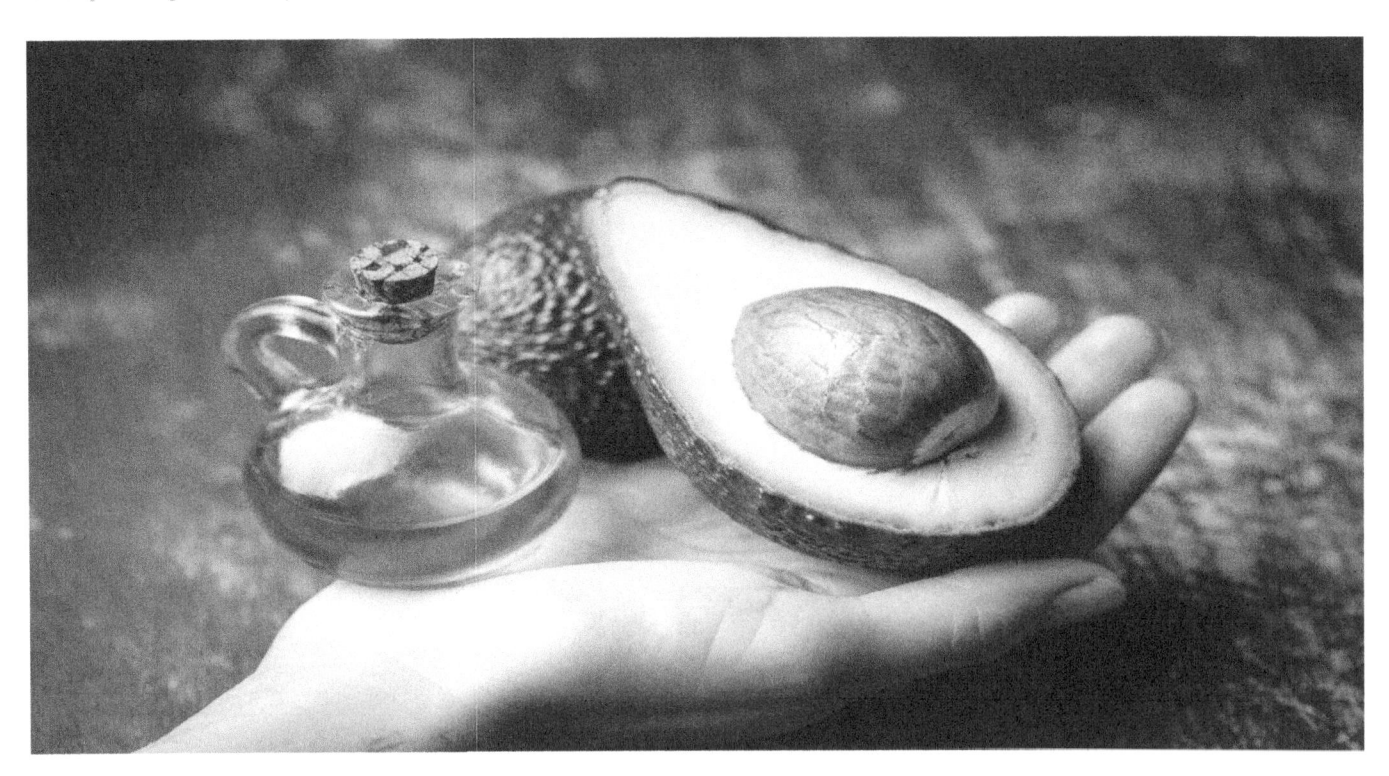

These recipes provide natural, gentle ways to care for the skin, combining the soothing and nourishing properties of ingredients like aloe vera, honey, tea tree, and oils. They can easily be adapted to suit individual skin needs, offering a balanced and holistic approach to skincare.

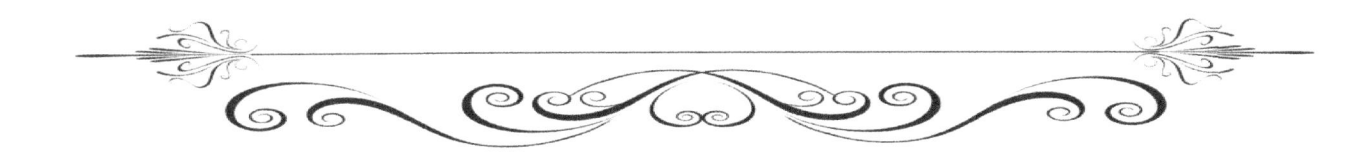

Chapter 6

Natural Remedies and Cardiovascular Health

The Contribution of Traditional Remedies: Garlic, Fish Oil, and Green Tea for Heart Health

Traditional remedies like garlic, fish oil, and green tea have long been used in various cultures to support cardiovascular health. Modern research has validated their heart-protective benefits, highlighting the potential of these natural ingredients to improve heart function, lower cholesterol, reduce inflammation, and support overall cardiovascular well-being. Here's a closer look at how these traditional remedies contribute to heart health:

Garlic: Nature's Heart Protector

Garlic (*Allium sativum*) has been used for centuries in natural medicine for its heart-health benefits. Packed with compounds like **allicin**—a sulfur compound released when garlic is crushed or chopped—garlic provides a range of protective effects for the cardiovascular system:

Reduces Blood Pressure: Studies show that garlic can help relax blood vessels and improve blood flow, leading to lower blood pressure. This effect is especially beneficial for individuals with hypertension, a key risk factor for heart disease.

Lowers Cholesterol Levels: Garlic has been found to reduce LDL ("bad") cholesterol while leaving HDL ("good") cholesterol levels largely unaffected. This helps maintain a healthy lipid profile and reduces the risk of plaque buildup in the arteries.

Prevents Blood Clotting: Garlic acts as a natural blood thinner, which may reduce the risk of clots that could lead to heart attacks or strokes.

How to Incorporate Garlic for Heart Health: Consuming fresh garlic or using garlic supplements standardized for allicin content can provide heart-health benefits. It is often recommended to consume 1-2 cloves of fresh garlic daily or take a standardized garlic supplement, as advised by a healthcare professional.

Fish Oil: Rich in Heart-Healthy Omega-3 Fatty Acids

Fish oil, derived from fatty fish like salmon, mackerel, and sardines, is rich in **omega-3 fatty acids**—particularly EPA (eicosapentaenoic acid) and DHA (docosahexaenoic acid). These essential fatty acids have been widely studied for their role in heart health and are known to provide several cardiovascular benefits:

Reduces Triglycerides: Omega-3s are known to lower triglyceride levels, which helps prevent atherosclerosis, or the buildup of fatty deposits in the arteries. Elevated triglycerides are a major risk factor for heart disease.

Lowers Blood Pressure: Omega-3s help relax blood vessels, leading to a reduction in blood pressure. They have a gentle blood-thinning effect, which may reduce the risk of blood clots.

Reduces Inflammation: Chronic inflammation is a contributing factor to cardiovascular disease. Omega-3 fatty acids possess anti-inflammatory properties that help reduce inflammation in blood vessels, supporting healthy artery function.

Improves Heart Rhythm: Omega-3s support a steady heart rhythm, which is particularly beneficial for individuals with arrhythmias or irregular heartbeats, reducing the risk of sudden cardiac events.

How to Incorporate Fish Oil for Heart Health: Fish oil supplements with high EPA and DHA content are widely available, or fish can be consumed directly. The American Heart Association recommends eating at least two servings of fatty fish per week, or taking a daily fish oil supplement of 1,000 mg EPA and DHA, though dosage may vary based on individual needs.

Green Tea: A Powerful Antioxidant for Cardiovascular Support

Green tea is known for its high concentration of **polyphenols**, especially **catechins** like EGCG (epigallocatechin gallate), which are potent antioxidants. These compounds play a significant role in protecting the heart by reducing oxidative stress and supporting healthy blood vessel function:

Reduces Cholesterol and Blood Pressure: Green tea catechins have been shown to lower LDL cholesterol levels and improve blood vessel flexibility, which can contribute to lower blood pressure and better circulation.

Improves Blood Vessel Function: Studies have shown that green tea helps maintain the integrity of blood vessel walls, promoting elasticity and reducing the likelihood of plaque formation.

Supports Weight Management: Green tea's catechins may support weight loss by boosting metabolism and fat oxidation. Maintaining a healthy weight is essential for reducing the risk of heart disease.

Reduces Inflammation: The anti-inflammatory properties of green tea help reduce damage to blood vessels caused by chronic inflammation, thus lowering the risk of developing cardiovascular issues.

How to Incorporate Green Tea for Heart Health: Drinking 2-3 cups of green tea daily can provide cardiovascular benefits. Green tea extracts, especially those standardized for catechin content, are also available as supplements for those who prefer a more concentrated source.

Integrating Garlic, Fish Oil, and Green Tea for Optimal Heart Health

Combining these three traditional remedies can provide comprehensive cardiovascular support. Garlic, fish oil, and green tea each bring unique benefits that, when combined, support heart health through different mechanisms:

Daily Routine: Incorporating fresh garlic into meals, drinking green tea, and supplementing with fish oil daily can form a simple, natural routine to promote heart health.

Complementary Effects: While fish oil primarily targets triglycerides and inflammation, garlic focuses on blood pressure and cholesterol, and green tea supports antioxidant protection and blood vessel health. Together, they create a well-rounded approach to heart care.

Lifestyle Considerations: Alongside these remedies, maintaining a balanced diet, regular physical activity, and stress management further enhances their heart-protective effects.

By using these natural remedies within a balanced lifestyle, it's possible to support cardiovascular function in a holistic, preventive way, utilizing the time-tested benefits of garlic, fish oil, and green tea for long-term heart health.

Modern Research on Cardiovascular Benefits: Studies Supporting the Effectiveness of These Remedies

Recent studies have provided compelling evidence to support the cardiovascular benefits of traditional remedies like garlic, fish oil, and green tea. Modern science has validated the long-standing use of these natural treatments by examining their effects on heart health, blood pressure, cholesterol, and inflammation. Here is a closer look at some key studies that demonstrate the heart-protective qualities of these remedies.

Garlic: Studies on Blood Pressure, Cholesterol, and Heart Health

Garlic's impact on cardiovascular health has been studied extensively, with research consistently showing its ability to support heart health by improving blood pressure, cholesterol, and reducing arterial plaque buildup:

Blood Pressure Reduction: A meta-analysis published in the *Journal of Clinical Hypertension* found that garlic supplementation significantly reduced systolic and diastolic blood pressure in people with hypertension. The study noted that participants taking garlic supplements experienced an average reduction of 6.7 mmHg in systolic and 4.8 mmHg in diastolic blood pressure, comparable to the effects of first-line antihypertensive drugs.

Cholesterol Lowering Effects: A study in *Nutrition Reviews* reviewed the cholesterol-lowering potential of garlic and concluded that garlic supplementation can reduce LDL ("bad") cholesterol by up to 10%. This is particularly beneficial for people at risk of cardiovascular disease, as lowering LDL levels helps prevent plaque buildup in the arteries.

Reduction of Arterial Plaque: Research published in *Atherosclerosis* demonstrated that garlic extracts could slow the progression of arterial plaque buildup, lowering the risk of atherosclerosis. The study suggested that garlic's anti-inflammatory and antioxidant effects contribute to improved artery health and circulation.

These findings confirm that regular garlic consumption, either in fresh form or as a supplement, has measurable benefits for cardiovascular health.

Fish Oil: Omega-3 Fatty Acids and Cardiovascular Protection

Fish oil, rich in omega-3 fatty acids (EPA and DHA), has been extensively researched for its heart health benefits. Studies have shown that omega-3s support the cardiovascular system by lowering triglycerides, reducing inflammation, and stabilizing heart rhythms:

Triglyceride Reduction: A comprehensive study published in the *Journal of the American Heart Association* revealed that fish oil supplements significantly reduce triglyceride levels, with high-dose omega-3 fatty acids leading to a reduction of up to 20-50% in triglyceride levels. High triglycerides are a known risk factor for heart disease, and this reduction is particularly beneficial for cardiovascular protection.

Anti-Inflammatory Effects: The *European Journal of Clinical Nutrition* published a study showing that omega-3 fatty acids in fish oil can reduce inflammatory markers like C-reactive protein (CRP) and interleukin-6. Reducing inflammation is crucial for preventing chronic cardiovascular issues, as inflammation contributes to arterial damage and plaque formation.

Improvement in Heart Rhythm: The *American Journal of Clinical Nutrition* reviewed studies on fish oil's effects on arrhythmias and concluded that omega-3 fatty acids help stabilize heart rhythms, reducing the likelihood of sudden cardiac death in individuals with heart disease.

The evidence from these studies highlights the role of omega-3s in fish oil as protective agents for heart health, reducing key cardiovascular risks through their anti-inflammatory, triglyceride-lowering, and heart rhythm-stabilizing properties.

Green Tea: Antioxidant-Rich Catechins and Heart Disease Prevention

Green tea, rich in catechins like EGCG, has demonstrated impressive cardiovascular benefits in multiple studies. These potent antioxidants help protect blood vessels, reduce oxidative stress, and improve blood lipid profiles, all of which contribute to heart health:

Cholesterol and Blood Pressure Benefits: A meta-analysis published in the *American Journal of Clinical Nutrition* reviewed multiple studies and concluded that green tea consumption significantly reduces LDL cholesterol levels and mildly lowers blood pressure. This dual benefit is essential for reducing the risk of atherosclerosis and improving circulation.

Blood Vessel Health and Flexibility: Research in the *Journal of Cardiovascular Pharmacology* explored the effects of green tea on vascular health. The study found that green tea catechins improve blood vessel elasticity and reduce arterial stiffness, key factors in maintaining healthy blood flow and reducing the risk of heart disease.

Reduced Oxidative Stress and Inflammation: A study published in *Free Radical Biology and Medicine* showed that green tea catechins effectively reduce oxidative stress in blood vessels. By protecting against oxidative damage, green tea helps reduce inflammation and slows the progression of cardiovascular disease.

The results of these studies validate green tea as a heart-protective beverage that supports blood vessel health, improves cholesterol levels, and provides antioxidant protection.

Combined Effects and Synergistic Benefits

Modern research also suggests that combining garlic, fish oil, and green tea could offer synergistic benefits for heart health. Each of these remedies addresses cardiovascular health through different mechanisms:

Garlic focuses on lowering blood pressure and improving cholesterol.
Fish Oil reduces triglycerides, inflammation, and supports heart rhythm.
Green Tea provides antioxidant protection and supports blood vessel elasticity.

Together, they create a well-rounded approach to cardiovascular wellness, each enhancing the effects of the others. This combination provides a comprehensive method for supporting heart health naturally, offering a multi-layered approach to protection against cardiovascular disease.

Scientific research has consistently supported the cardiovascular benefits of garlic, fish oil, and green tea. These natural remedies, used for centuries, are now validated by studies showing their effectiveness in lowering blood pressure, reducing cholesterol and triglycerides, combating inflammation, and protecting blood vessels. By incorporating these traditional remedies, individuals can create a well-supported, heart-healthy routine, bridging ancient wisdom with modern science for optimal cardiovascular wellness.

Integrated Strategies for Heart Health: Combining Natural Remedies with Lifestyle Management and Medications, When Necessary

Maintaining optimal heart health requires a well-rounded approach that combines natural remedies, lifestyle adjustments, and, when needed, medications. Natural ingredients like garlic, fish oil, and green tea offer significant cardiovascular benefits, but they work best when incorporated alongside heart-healthy lifestyle changes, such as diet, exercise, and stress management. For individuals with existing cardiovascular conditions, medications may also be essential. Here's a guide on how to combine these elements to create a comprehensive, integrated strategy for heart health.

Natural Remedies for Heart Health

Using Garlic, Fish Oil, and Green Tea:
Garlic: Known for its ability to reduce blood pressure, cholesterol, and inflammation, garlic can be easily added to meals or taken as a supplement. Fresh garlic cloves, garlic oil, or garlic extract capsules are all effective ways to incorporate garlic into a daily routine.
Fish Oil: High in omega-3 fatty acids, fish oil supplements can help lower triglycerides and reduce inflammation, both of which are important for heart health. The American Heart Association recommends 1,000 mg of EPA and DHA daily, although higher doses may be recommended by healthcare providers for individuals with high triglycerides.

Green Tea: Drinking 2-3 cups of green tea daily can contribute antioxidants that help protect blood vessels, lower LDL cholesterol, and improve circulation. Green tea supplements can also be an option for those who prefer a concentrated form.

Combining Remedies for Synergy: Each of these remedies has unique cardiovascular benefits, and using them together can provide a more comprehensive approach. For example, garlic's cholesterol-lowering effects complement fish oil's triglyceride-reducing effects, while green tea provides additional antioxidant support.

Lifestyle Adjustments for Optimal Heart Health

Nutrition:

Adopt a Heart-Healthy Diet: A balanced diet, rich in whole grains, lean proteins, and healthy fats, is essential for cardiovascular health. The Mediterranean diet, for instance, emphasizes olive oil, fish, vegetables, and whole grains and is associated with a lower risk of heart disease.

Limit Sodium Intake: Excessive sodium can elevate blood pressure, so it's important to limit intake to less than 2,300 mg per day, or ideally around 1,500 mg for those at risk.

Increase Fiber and Antioxidants: Foods high in fiber, such as fruits, vegetables, and whole grains, can help lower cholesterol levels. Antioxidant-rich foods, like berries and leafy greens, reduce oxidative stress, benefiting heart health.

Physical Activity:

Exercise Regularly: Physical activity strengthens the heart and improves circulation. Aim for at least 150 minutes of moderate exercise or 75 minutes of vigorous exercise per week. Activities like brisk walking, cycling, and swimming are particularly beneficial for cardiovascular health.

Incorporate Strength Training: Resistance exercises, performed 2-3 times a week, complement cardiovascular activity by building muscle, improving metabolic function, and supporting overall heart health.

Stress Management:

Practice Mindfulness and Relaxation Techniques: Chronic stress can raise blood pressure and trigger inflammatory responses, which harm the heart. Mindfulness practices like meditation, deep breathing exercises, and yoga can reduce stress and improve mental resilience.

Establish a Consistent Sleep Routine: Quality sleep allows the heart to recover and helps regulate blood pressure. Aim for 7-9 hours of sleep per night to maintain healthy heart function.

When Medications are Necessary

For individuals with diagnosed heart conditions, medications may be an essential part of their heart health plan. It is possible to integrate natural remedies and lifestyle changes with prescribed medications effectively, but it's crucial to do so under medical supervision:

Common Heart Medications and How They Work:

Statins: These are prescribed to lower LDL cholesterol, reducing the risk of atherosclerosis and heart attacks. Some studies suggest that garlic may have a mild cholesterol-lowering effect, but it is not a substitute for statins in people with high cholesterol.

Antihypertensives: Medications like ACE inhibitors and beta-blockers help control high blood pressure. Garlic's natural blood pressure-lowering properties can complement these medications but should be monitored to prevent blood pressure from dropping too low.
Anticoagulants: Blood thinners, such as warfarin, prevent blood clots. Since garlic and fish oil both have mild blood-thinning properties, it's important to consult a healthcare provider to avoid excessive thinning.
Integrating Medications with Natural Remedies:
Monitor Dosages: If you are using both natural remedies and prescription medications, follow the recommended dosages closely and consult your doctor to prevent interactions or excessive effects.
Track Your Heart Health Markers: Regularly check blood pressure, cholesterol levels, and triglycerides to understand how natural remedies and medications are affecting you. This will help you and your healthcare provider make necessary adjustments.
Communicate with Your Healthcare Provider: Let your healthcare provider know about any supplements or natural remedies you're taking to ensure there are no contraindications with prescribed medications.

Building a Personalized Heart Health Plan

An integrated approach to heart health requires careful planning and consistency. Here are some steps to create a personalized plan:
Step 1: Assess Your Health Status: Begin by consulting with a healthcare provider to assess your current heart health, including cholesterol levels, blood pressure, triglycerides, and inflammation markers.
Step 2: Set Realistic Goals: Set clear, achievable goals for your heart health. These could include reducing cholesterol, lowering blood pressure, or improving physical fitness. Make sure these goals align with both natural and medical treatments as needed.
Step 3: Create a Balanced Routine: Develop a daily routine that includes heart-healthy foods, regular exercise, and natural remedies like garlic, fish oil, and green tea. Incorporate stress management techniques and prioritize quality sleep.
Step 4: Monitor Progress: Track your progress through regular check-ups, lab work, and by noting any changes in your energy levels or well-being. Adjust your routine as needed based on your results.
Step 5: Adapt as Needed: If your health changes, or if your body needs additional support, don't hesitate to consult your healthcare provider about modifying your routine, adjusting medication dosages, or introducing new remedies.

An integrated strategy for heart health, combining natural remedies, lifestyle modifications, and, when needed, medications, offers a comprehensive approach to cardiovascular wellness. By incorporating traditional remedies like garlic, fish oil, and green tea, alongside dietary improvements, regular exercise, and effective stress management, you can create a balanced, heart-healthy routine. Always work closely with a healthcare provider to ensure your approach is safe and effective, and embrace a proactive role in managing your heart health for long-term wellness.

Heart-Healthy Recipes: Teas, Juices, and Dishes with Traditional Ingredients Like Garlic, Green Tea, and Fish Oil

This collection of 25 heart-healthy recipes combines the time-tested benefits of traditional ingredients such as garlic, green tea, and fish oil with delicious, easy-to-make teas, juices, and dishes. Each recipe is crafted to support cardiovascular health by promoting better circulation, reducing inflammation, and maintaining healthy cholesterol and blood pressure levels. From soothing teas and antioxidant-rich juices to flavorful dishes, these recipes are designed to enhance heart health while incorporating wholesome, natural flavors.

These recipes offer a well-rounded approach to heart wellness, using the powerful properties of natural ingredients to create meals and beverages that are as enjoyable as they are beneficial. Perfect for those looking to integrate heart-friendly practices into their daily diet, this collection provides a flavorful pathway to improved cardiovascular health.

25 recipes for the well-being of the heart

101. Garlic & Lemon Heart Tonic

Description: A refreshing tonic to support circulation and heart health.
Ingredients:
- 1 clove **garlic**, minced
- Juice of 1/2 **lemon**
- 1 cup warm water

Instructions:
- Mix minced garlic and lemon juice with warm water.
- Stir well and consume on an empty stomach in the morning.

Variation:
- **Add Honey**: Add 1 tsp honey for a smoother taste and additional antibacterial benefits.

How to Use: Drink daily in the morning for optimal benefits.

102. Green Tea & Ginger Anti-Inflammatory Tea

Description: A warm tea rich in antioxidants to reduce inflammation and support the heart.
Ingredients:
- 1 cup hot water
- 1 **green tea bag**
- 1/2 tsp grated **ginger**

Instructions:
- Steep green tea bag and grated ginger in hot water for 5-7 minutes.
- Strain and sip slowly.

Variation:
- **Add Lemon**: Squeeze in lemon juice for additional vitamin C.

How to Use: Drink 1-2 times daily, ideally after meals.

103. Spinach & Fish Oil Smoothie

Description: A nutrient-dense smoothie loaded with heart-supportive omega-3s.
Ingredients:
- 1 cup **spinach**
- 1/2 cup **apple juice**
- 1 **fish oil capsule** (open and add liquid content)

Instructions:
- Blend spinach, apple juice, and fish oil until smooth.
- Consume immediately for maximum nutrient retention.

Variation:
- **Add Banana**: Add 1/2 banana for a touch of sweetness and added potassium.

How to Use: Enjoy 3-4 times per week as a snack or part of breakfast.

---

104. Garlic & Olive Oil Roasted Vegetables

Description: A delicious side dish packed with heart-healthy garlic and olive oil.
Ingredients:
- 1 cup chopped **broccoli**
- 1 cup chopped **carrots**
- 3 cloves **garlic**, minced
- 2 tbsp **olive oil**

Instructions:
- Preheat oven to 400°F (200°C).
- Toss vegetables with garlic and olive oil.
- Spread on a baking sheet and roast for 20-25 minutes.

How to Use: Serve as a side dish with meals, 2-3 times a week.

---

105. Heart-Boosting Green Juice

Description: A fresh juice to detoxify and support cardiovascular health.
Ingredients:
- 1 cup **spinach**
- 1/2 **cucumber**
- 1 **green apple**
- 1/2 tsp **grated ginger**

Instructions:
- Juice all ingredients in a juicer.
- Stir well and enjoy immediately.

How to Use: Drink in the morning to start the day with antioxidants and detoxifying nutrients.

---

106. Omega-3 Fish Oil Salad Dressing

Description: A simple salad dressing infused with fish oil for a boost of omega-3s.
Ingredients:
- 1 tbsp **olive oil**
- 1/2 tsp **fish oil** (or contents of 1 capsule)
- 1 tsp **lemon juice**
- Salt and pepper to taste

Instructions:
- Mix olive oil, fish oil, and lemon juice until well blended.
- Drizzle over salads.

How to Use: Use with salads 2-3 times a week.

107. Garlic & Spinach Sauté

Description: A quick and heart-friendly dish with garlic and spinach.
Ingredients:
- 2 cups **fresh spinach**
- 2 cloves **garlic**, minced
- 1 tbsp **olive oil**

Instructions:
- Heat olive oil in a pan, add garlic and sauté until fragrant.
- Add spinach, cook until wilted.

How to Use: Serve as a side dish or with whole grains; enjoy 2-3 times per week.

---

108. Green Tea & Mint Iced Tea

Description: A refreshing iced tea with antioxidants for heart support.
Ingredients:
- 2 cups brewed **green tea**
- 5-6 fresh **mint leaves**
- 1 tsp **honey** (optional)

Instructions:
- Brew green tea, let it cool, and add mint leaves.
- Add honey if desired, pour over ice.

How to Use: Enjoy once daily for antioxidant support.

---

109. Garlic & Herb Baked Salmon

Description: A heart-healthy salmon dish rich in omega-3 fatty acids.
Ingredients:
- 1 salmon fillet
- 2 cloves **garlic**, minced
- 1 tsp **olive oil**
- Fresh herbs (thyme or rosemary)

Instructions:
- Preheat oven to 375°F (190°C).
- Rub garlic, olive oil, and herbs over salmon.
- Bake for 15-20 minutes until flaky.

How to Use: Enjoy as a main course 1-2 times per week.

---

110. Beet & Berry Heart-Healthy Smoothie

Description: A nutrient-packed smoothie for better blood flow and heart health.
Ingredients:
- 1 small **beet**, cooked and chopped
- 1/2 cup **blueberries**
- 1/2 cup **unsweetened almond milk**

Instructions:
- Blend all ingredients until smooth.

How to Use: Enjoy as a morning or afternoon snack, 2-3 times per week.

111. Garlic & Lemon Chickpea Salad

Description: A filling salad with heart-friendly ingredients.
Ingredients:
- 1 can **chickpeas**, drained and rinsed
- 1 clove **garlic**, minced
- Juice of 1 **lemon**
- 1 tbsp **olive oil**

Instructions:
- Mix chickpeas, garlic, lemon juice, and olive oil.
- Toss to coat.

How to Use: Serve as a main or side dish, 2-3 times per week.

---

112. Green Tea Smoothie Bowl

Description: A creamy smoothie bowl packed with antioxidants.
Ingredients:
- 1 cup brewed **green tea**, cooled
- 1/2 **banana**
- 1/4 cup **spinach**

Instructions:
- Blend all ingredients and pour into a bowl.
- Top with fresh fruit or nuts.

How to Use: Ideal for breakfast or a light lunch.

---

113. Cucumber & Mint Green Tea

Description: A refreshing beverage for hydration and heart health.
Ingredients:
- 1 cup brewed **green tea**, cooled
- 4 slices **cucumber**
- 5 fresh **mint leaves**

Instructions:
- Add cucumber and mint to green tea, refrigerate until cold.

How to Use: Enjoy any time of day.

---

114. Garlic & Olive Oil Dip

Description: A heart-healthy dip for bread or vegetables.
Ingredients:
- 1/4 cup **olive oil**
- 2 cloves **garlic**, minced
- 1/2 tsp dried **oregano**

Instructions:
- Mix all ingredients and serve with whole grain bread or vegetables.

How to Use: Use as a dipping sauce.

115. Turmeric & Ginger Heart-Healthy Latte

Description: A warm, antioxidant-rich drink for heart health.
Ingredients:
- 1 cup **almond milk**
- 1/2 tsp **turmeric**
- 1/2 tsp grated **ginger**

Instructions:
Heat almond milk, then stir in turmeric and ginger.
How to Use: Enjoy in the evening for relaxation.

---

116. Garlic, Tomato & Basil Bruschetta

Description: A flavorful heart-friendly appetizer rich in antioxidants.
Ingredients:
- 1 cup **cherry tomatoes**, diced
- 2 cloves **garlic**, minced
- 1 tbsp **olive oil**
- Fresh **basil** leaves, chopped
- Whole grain baguette slices

Instructions:
Mix tomatoes, garlic, olive oil, and basil.
Spoon mixture onto toasted baguette slices.
How to Use: Enjoy as a light appetizer or snack, 2-3 times per week.

---

117. Lemon & Green Tea Heart Tonic

Description: A refreshing, heart-protective tonic loaded with antioxidants.
Ingredients:
- 1 cup brewed **green tea**, cooled
- Juice of 1 **lemon**
- 1 tsp **honey** (optional)

Instructions:
Mix green tea with lemon juice and honey.
Stir well and enjoy over ice.
How to Use: Drink daily in the morning or early afternoon.

---

118. Omega-3 Enriched Avocado Toast

Description: A heart-healthy breakfast option with healthy fats.
Ingredients:
- 1 slice **whole grain bread**
- 1/2 **avocado**, mashed
- 1 **fish oil capsule** (optional, contents only)

Instructions:
Spread mashed avocado on toast.
Open fish oil capsule and mix in for extra omega-3s.
How to Use: Enjoy for breakfast 3-4 times a week.

119. Garlic & Lemon Salmon

Description: A main dish rich in omega-3s for cardiovascular health.
Ingredients:
- 1 salmon fillet
- 2 cloves **garlic**, minced
- Juice of 1/2 **lemon**
- 1 tsp **olive oil**

Instructions:
- Preheat oven to 375°F (190°C).
- Place garlic and lemon juice on salmon, drizzle with olive oil.
- Bake for 15-20 minutes until cooked.

How to Use: Enjoy once a week as a main dish.

---

120. Pomegranate & Berry Heart-Healthy Smoothie

Description: A smoothie packed with antioxidants for heart protection.
Ingredients:
- 1/2 cup **pomegranate juice**
- 1/2 cup **mixed berries**
- 1/4 cup **spinach**

Instructions:
- Blend all ingredients until smooth.

How to Use: Drink in the morning or as a snack, 3-4 times a week.

---

121. Garlic & Herb Olive Oil Spread

Description: A heart-healthy spread for sandwiches or dipping.
Ingredients:
- 1/4 cup **olive oil**
- 3 cloves **garlic**, minced
- 1/2 tsp dried **rosemary**

Instructions:
- Combine ingredients and let sit for 10-15 minutes to infuse.

How to Use: Use as a spread or dip with whole grain bread, 2-3 times per week.

---

122. Green Tea & Berry Infused Water

Description: A refreshing drink to boost hydration and heart health.
Ingredients:
- 1 cup brewed **green tea**, cooled
- 1/4 cup **fresh berries**
- 5-6 fresh **mint leaves**

Instructions:
- Add berries and mint to green tea.
- Refrigerate for 1-2 hours before drinking.

How to Use: Enjoy throughout the day as a hydrating, antioxidant-rich beverage.

123. Garlic & Avocado Salad Dressing

Description: A creamy, heart-healthy dressing for salads.
Ingredients:
- 1/2 **avocado**, mashed
- 1 clove **garlic**, minced
- Juice of 1/2 **lemon**

Instructions:
Blend all ingredients until smooth and creamy.
How to Use: Drizzle over salads 2-3 times per week.

---

124. Turmeric & Green Tea Latte

Description: A warm latte with heart-protective turmeric and green tea.
Ingredients:
- 1 cup brewed **green tea**
- 1/2 tsp **turmeric powder**
- 1 tsp **honey** (optional)

Instructions:
Mix turmeric into warm green tea and add honey if desired.
How to Use: Enjoy as a mid-morning or afternoon drink, daily

---

125. Omega-3 Rich Chia Pudding

Description: A heart-healthy dessert rich in omega-3s.
Ingredients:
- 1 cup **almond milk**
- 3 tbsp **chia seeds**
- 1/2 tsp **vanilla extract**

Instructions:
Mix all ingredients and refrigerate for at least 2 hours or overnight.
How to Use: Enjoy as a snack or dessert 2-3 times per week.

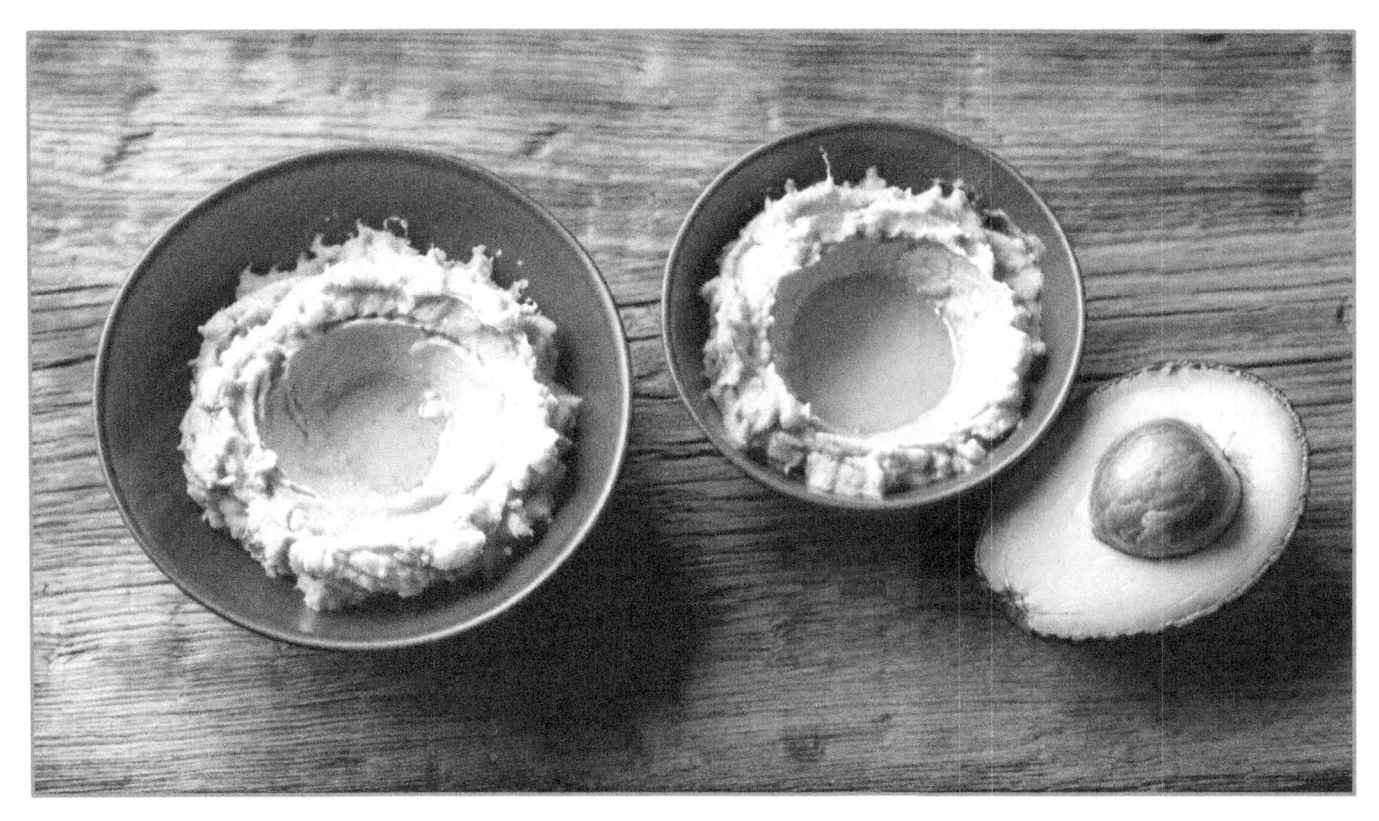

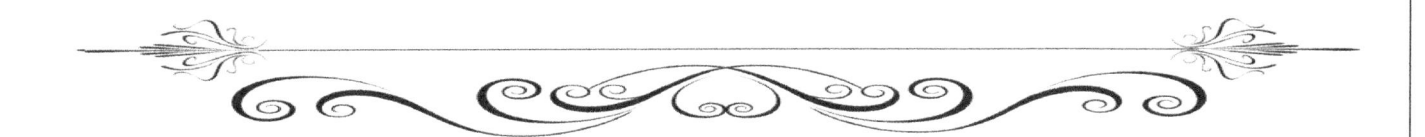

Chapter 7

Energy Management and General Welfare

Remedies for Energy and Wellness: Ginseng, Ashwagandha, and Other Adaptogenic Herbs

Adaptogenic herbs like ginseng, ashwagandha, and others are renowned for their ability to enhance energy, reduce stress, and promote overall wellness. These herbs help the body adapt to physical and mental stress by balancing cortisol levels, improving resilience, and enhancing mental clarity. Adaptogens have been used for centuries in traditional medicine systems, such as Ayurveda and Traditional Chinese Medicine (TCM), for their powerful effects on vitality and stress reduction. Here's an in-depth look at the top adaptogenic herbs and how they can be incorporated into a routine to boost energy and support well-being.

Ginseng: The Vitality Herb

Ginseng, particularly **Panax ginseng** (Asian ginseng) and **Panax quinquefolius** (American ginseng), is widely used for its ability to enhance energy, reduce fatigue, and improve mental focus. Ginseng's active compounds, known as **ginsenosides**, support the adrenal glands, which play a crucial role in stress response and energy production. Key benefits of ginseng include:

Increased Physical Stamina: Ginseng is known to reduce fatigue and boost endurance, making it a popular choice for those looking to increase physical performance.

Enhanced Mental Clarity: Studies have shown that ginseng improves cognitive function and focus, which is beneficial for managing mental stress.

Immune System Support: Ginseng helps support the immune system, making it an ideal herb for overall health maintenance.

How to Use Ginseng: Ginseng is available in various forms, including capsules, powders, and teas. It's best taken in the morning to prevent any potential interference with sleep, as it can be energizing. Typical doses range from 200-400 mg of standardized extract daily, but always consult with a healthcare provider for personalized guidance.

Ashwagandha: The Stress-Relieving Adaptogen

Ashwagandha (**Withania somnifera**) is a powerful adaptogen used in Ayurveda for centuries to reduce stress and anxiety, improve energy levels, and enhance mood. Known as the "strength of the stallion," ashwagandha is renowned for its ability to increase endurance and vitality. The key benefits of ashwagandha include:

Reduced Cortisol Levels: Studies have shown that ashwagandha can reduce cortisol, the stress hormone, helping the body manage daily stress more effectively.

Improved Sleep and Relaxation: Ashwagandha promotes better sleep quality and relaxation, making it a great choice for those struggling with anxiety or insomnia.

Increased Physical Strength and Endurance: Athletes often use ashwagandha to improve stamina and reduce exercise-induced muscle damage.

How to Use Ashwagandha: Ashwagandha is available as a powder, capsule, or tincture. It can be taken in the morning or evening, depending on individual needs, as it has both energizing and calming effects. A common dose is 300-600 mg of standardized extract daily. Many people enjoy ashwagandha powder in warm milk or smoothies.

Rhodiola Rosea: The Endurance Enhancer

Rhodiola rosea, also known as "golden root," is an adaptogenic herb commonly used to enhance endurance, reduce fatigue, and improve mood. Rhodiola is particularly effective in helping the body cope with physical and mental stress by supporting the nervous system and promoting resilience. The benefits of Rhodiola rosea include:

Enhanced Physical Endurance: Rhodiola helps improve stamina and endurance, making it a popular choice for athletes and active individuals.

Improved Mood and Reduced Anxiety: Rhodiola has been shown to reduce symptoms of depression and anxiety by supporting neurotransmitter balance.

Better Mental Clarity and Focus: Rhodiola improves cognitive function, concentration, and overall mental performance.

How to Use Rhodiola Rosea: Rhodiola is most commonly available in capsule or tincture form. It's typically taken in doses of 200-400 mg per day, and it's best consumed in the morning or early afternoon to avoid potential sleep disturbances.

Holy Basil: The Calming Herb

Holy basil (**Ocimum sanctum**), also known as "tulsi," is revered in Ayurveda as a sacred plant with remarkable adaptogenic properties. Known for its calming effects, holy basil supports the body's response to stress and promotes a sense of well-being and balance. Key benefits of holy basil include:

Reduced Anxiety and Stress: Holy basil helps balance cortisol levels, which can reduce stress and promote relaxation.

Antioxidant Protection: Rich in antioxidants, holy basil helps protect the body from oxidative stress and supports overall immune health.

Enhanced Mental Clarity: Holy basil supports cognitive function and focus, making it an excellent choice for those facing mental stress.

How to Use Holy Basil: Holy basil is available as a tea, capsule, or tincture. Many people enjoy holy basil tea daily as a soothing ritual. Typical doses range from 400-600 mg per day, and it can be taken at any time of the day.

Maca Root: The Energizing Root

Maca root (**Lepidium meyenii**), native to Peru, is commonly used for its ability to increase energy, improve mood, and support hormonal balance. Maca is especially beneficial for individuals who experience fatigue related to hormonal imbalances or low energy. The benefits of maca root include:

Increased Energy and Stamina: Maca is known to enhance physical endurance and reduce feelings of fatigue, making it popular among athletes and active individuals.

Enhanced Mood and Mental Clarity: Maca has adaptogenic properties that support emotional balance and mental well-being.

Hormone Balance: Maca helps regulate hormones, particularly in women, providing relief from PMS and menopause symptoms.

How to Use Maca Root: Maca powder can be added to smoothies, oatmeal, or coffee. Typical doses range from 1-3 grams per day, and it's best consumed in the morning for an energy boost throughout the day.

Eleuthero: The Energy-Boosting Herb

Eleuthero (**Eleutherococcus senticosus**), also known as Siberian ginseng, is an adaptogen used in Traditional Chinese Medicine to improve physical and mental stamina. Eleuthero is commonly used to increase energy, reduce fatigue, and support immune health. Key benefits of eleuthero include:

Enhanced Physical and Mental Endurance: Eleuthero improves stamina, making it beneficial for those who need sustained energy throughout the day.

Stress Relief: Eleuthero helps balance cortisol levels, reducing the impact of stress on the body.

Immune System Support: Eleuthero supports immune function, helping the body resist illness.

How to Use Eleuthero: Eleuthero is available in capsules, powders, and tinctures. A typical daily dose ranges from 300-600 mg, and it's best taken in the morning.

Combining Adaptogens for Optimal Energy and Wellness

Combining these adaptogenic herbs can provide a well-rounded approach to boosting energy, improving resilience to stress, and enhancing overall well-being. Here are some strategies for incorporating multiple adaptogens into a routine:

Morning Blend: A combination of ginseng, maca, and eleuthero can provide an energizing start to the day. Blend them into a smoothie or take them in capsule form.

Evening Calm: Holy basil and ashwagandha taken in the evening can promote relaxation and improve sleep quality.

Workout Support: Rhodiola and maca are excellent for pre-workout energy and endurance. They can be taken 30-60 minutes before exercise to reduce fatigue.

Precautions and Tips

Consult a Healthcare Provider: While adaptogens are generally safe, it's best to consult a healthcare provider if you are pregnant, breastfeeding, or taking medications, as some adaptogens may interact with certain drugs.

Start Slowly: Begin with lower doses to assess how your body responds, gradually increasing as needed.

Cycle Your Adaptogens: To prevent tolerance, consider cycling adaptogens by using them for 6-8 weeks, followed by a break of 1-2 weeks.

Adaptogenic herbs like ginseng, ashwagandha, and others provide a natural, holistic way to support energy, reduce stress, and promote overall well-being. By integrating these herbs into your daily routine, you can enjoy increased vitality, mental clarity, and resilience to the demands of modern life.

Support from Modern Medicine: How Recent Studies Have Uncovered Mechanisms of Action and Enhanced the Safety of These Supplements

Modern medicine has provided valuable insights into how adaptogenic supplements like ginseng, ashwagandha, and other traditional herbs impact the body at a molecular level. Through recent scientific studies, researchers have identified the specific mechanisms of action that make these supplements effective for supporting energy, reducing stress, and enhancing overall well-being. Moreover, advances in research and technology have improved the safety and efficacy of these natural remedies, allowing for better quality control, accurate dosages, and optimized formulations. Here's a closer look at the breakthroughs in understanding these supplements and how modern medicine has enhanced their safety for consumers.

Mechanisms of Action: Understanding How Adaptogens Work

Recent research has clarified how adaptogens exert their effects by interacting with the body's stress-response systems, hormonal pathways, and energy production. Here are some of the mechanisms identified:

Regulating the Hypothalamic-Pituitary-Adrenal (HPA) Axis: Many adaptogens, including ashwagandha and rhodiola, help modulate the HPA axis—a central component of the body's stress response. By balancing cortisol levels and reducing excess production of stress hormones, adaptogens help the body respond to physical and mental stress without overwhelming the system.

Supporting Neurotransmitter Balance: Adaptogens like ginseng and rhodiola have been shown to influence key neurotransmitters, such as dopamine, serotonin, and norepinephrine. This action helps to improve mood, reduce anxiety, and enhance mental clarity. For example, rhodiola's effects on serotonin and dopamine are thought to be responsible for its mood-enhancing properties, making it beneficial for those facing stress-related mood imbalances.

Reducing Oxidative Stress and Inflammation: Oxidative stress and inflammation are contributors to chronic health issues, including fatigue and mental exhaustion. Adaptogens such as holy basil and ginseng are rich in antioxidants, which protect cells from damage caused by free radicals. Studies have shown that these antioxidants help reduce markers of inflammation, thus protecting cells and tissues from stress-related damage.

Enhancing Mitochondrial Function: The mitochondria, the energy powerhouses of cells, play a key role in energy production. Adaptogens like maca and ashwagandha have been found to enhance mitochondrial function, thereby increasing energy production and stamina at the cellular level. This mechanism is particularly beneficial for reducing physical fatigue and improving endurance.

These discoveries have validated the traditional uses of adaptogens and provided a scientific basis for their benefits, making them more accepted and integrated into modern wellness practices.

Improved Safety and Quality Control in Adaptogenic Supplements

Modern scientific advances have also led to significant improvements in the safety and quality of adaptogenic supplements. In the past, inconsistent formulations and purity concerns sometimes impacted the effectiveness and safety of herbal supplements. Today, rigorous testing standards and enhanced extraction techniques have greatly improved the quality and reliability of these products. Some of these improvements include:

Standardized Extracts for Consistent Dosages: Standardization involves isolating and quantifying the active compounds in adaptogenic herbs, such as ginsenosides in ginseng or withanolides in ashwagandha. This standardization ensures that each supplement contains a precise amount of active ingredients, making dosage more accurate and consistent. Standardized extracts are safer and more effective because they reduce variability in potency.

Third-Party Testing for Purity and Safety: Many reputable brands now employ third-party testing to verify the purity and quality of their supplements. These tests check for contaminants like heavy metals, pesticides, and microbes, which can sometimes be present in natural products. Ensuring purity is particularly important for long-term health and safety, as contaminants can accumulate in the body over time.

Advanced Extraction Techniques: Improved extraction methods, such as CO_2 extraction, produce cleaner, more potent extracts without the use of harsh chemicals. These methods allow for a higher concentration of active compounds, resulting in more effective products that are free from potentially harmful solvents.

Research-Backed Dosage Recommendations: Recent studies have established recommended dosages for many adaptogens, making it easier to use these supplements safely and effectively. For instance, studies on ashwagandha have found that doses of 300-600 mg of standardized extract are effective for reducing stress and improving energy levels. This research-backed dosing helps consumers avoid excessive use, which can sometimes lead to unwanted side effects.

Clinical Studies Supporting the Safety of Adaptogens

Clinical trials on adaptogens have highlighted their safety profiles and provided insight into potential side effects and interactions, allowing for more informed use. Some of the findings from recent studies include:

Minimal Side Effects with Proper Dosing: Studies on popular adaptogens like ashwagandha and rhodiola have shown that, when taken within the recommended dosage ranges, they have minimal side effects. Ashwagandha, for example, is generally well tolerated and has been shown to reduce stress with few adverse effects. However, very high doses may cause gastrointestinal discomfort, underscoring the importance of following dosage guidelines.

Understanding Potential Interactions: Research has highlighted that some adaptogens may interact with specific medications. For example, ginseng can potentially interact with blood-thinning medications due to its mild anticoagulant properties. As a result, healthcare providers can better advise on adaptogen use alongside medications, enhancing safety.

Improved Formulations for Enhanced Absorption: Some studies have focused on improving bioavailability—the rate at which the body absorbs a substance. Adaptogens like ashwagandha and ginseng are now often combined with other ingredients, such as black pepper extract (piperine), to enhance absorption and maximize effectiveness. These formulations allow for lower doses while maintaining efficacy, further reducing the risk of side effects.

Integrating Adaptogens Safely into Modern Health Practices

As adaptogens become more popular in modern wellness routines, healthcare providers and wellness practitioners are increasingly recommending them as part of a balanced approach to health. Some considerations for safe and effective use include:

Personalized Recommendations: Healthcare providers can now make personalized recommendations based on individual health profiles, stress levels, and wellness goals. For example, an individual with high stress may benefit from ashwagandha for its calming effects, while an athlete might benefit more from rhodiola for enhanced endurance.

Guidelines for Cycling and Rotation: To prevent the body from becoming accustomed to a single adaptogen, some practitioners recommend cycling or rotating adaptogens. For instance, one could take ashwagandha for 8 weeks, then switch to rhodiola for another 8 weeks. Cycling helps maintain the effectiveness of adaptogens over time.

Combining with Other Supplements for Synergy: Modern formulations sometimes combine adaptogens with vitamins, minerals, or other herbs to enhance their effects. Adaptogens are often paired with B vitamins, which support energy metabolism, or magnesium, which further aids in stress reduction. These synergies provide comprehensive support for energy, mental clarity, and resilience.

Modern research has illuminated the mechanisms by which adaptogenic herbs like ginseng, ashwagandha, and rhodiola support energy, reduce stress, and promote wellness. Advances in quality control, standardized dosages, and purity testing have made these supplements safer and more reliable, allowing consumers to benefit from their potent effects with greater confidence. As adaptogens continue to gain popularity in the wellness world, their integration into evidence-based healthcare practices has enhanced both their efficacy and safety, making them a trusted ally for natural stress relief, energy, and overall well-being.

Practical Tips for Integration: How to Choose the Best Products and Combine Them with Modern Lifestyle Strategies

Incorporating adaptogens and other natural supplements into a wellness routine can be highly beneficial, but choosing the right products and combining them with healthy lifestyle practices is key to maximizing their effects. With the wide variety of products available today, it's important to understand how to select high-quality supplements and integrate them effectively into a balanced lifestyle. Here are some practical tips to guide you in selecting the best adaptogenic products and pairing them with modern strategies for stress reduction, energy, and overall wellness.

Choosing High-Quality Adaptogenic Products

Look for Standardized Extracts: When choosing adaptogenic herbs like ginseng, ashwagandha, or rhodiola, opt for standardized extracts. Standardization ensures that each dose contains a consistent amount of active compounds, such as ginsenosides in ginseng or withanolides in ashwagandha, which are responsible for the herb's effects. Products that list these percentages (e.g., "contains 5% withanolides") provide a more reliable, effective dose.

Check for Third-Party Testing: Reputable brands often use third-party testing to verify the purity and potency of their supplements. Look for products that display certification from independent testing organizations, as this indicates that they have been tested for contaminants, such as heavy metals, pesticides, and microbes. Ensuring purity is especially important for long-term safety and effectiveness.

Choose Organic and Sustainably Sourced Options: Whenever possible, select organic and sustainably sourced adaptogens. Organic products are grown without synthetic pesticides and chemicals, and sustainable sourcing helps preserve the ecosystems where these herbs are cultivated. Some adaptogens, like rhodiola and ashwagandha, are especially vulnerable to environmental overharvesting, so choosing sustainably sourced options can help support environmental health.

Consider the Form of the Supplement: Adaptogens are available in various forms, including powders, capsules, tinctures, and teas. Choose a form that fits your lifestyle and is easy to integrate into your routine:

Capsules are convenient for precise dosing and are ideal for people with busy lifestyles.

Powders are versatile and can be added to smoothies, coffee, or water.

Tinctures offer quick absorption and can be taken in small, customizable doses.

Combining Adaptogens with Modern Lifestyle Practices

Pair with a Balanced Diet: Adaptogens work best when supported by a nutrient-dense diet. A diet rich in whole foods—such as leafy greens, lean proteins, healthy fats, and complex carbohydrates—ensures that your body has the vitamins and minerals needed to process and utilize adaptogens effectively. Key nutrients like B vitamins, magnesium, and antioxidants enhance the stress-reducing and energy-boosting effects of adaptogens. Additionally, eating balanced meals stabilizes blood sugar levels, which can further support sustained energy.

Use Adaptogens to Complement Physical Activity: Physical activity plays a significant role in managing stress and boosting energy levels. Adaptogens like rhodiola and maca are excellent pre-workout supplements because they increase stamina and reduce fatigue, making them beneficial for both endurance and strength training. For post-workout recovery, ashwagandha and holy basil help reduce inflammation and speed up muscle repair.

Pre-Workout Routine: Take rhodiola or maca 30 minutes before exercising to improve endurance.

Post-Workout Recovery: Consider a small dose of ashwagandha or holy basil after exercise to support muscle recovery and reduce stress.

Incorporate Adaptogens into a Sleep Routine: Quality sleep is essential for overall wellness and helps the body better manage stress. Adaptogens like ashwagandha and holy basil promote relaxation and are ideal additions to an evening routine to improve sleep quality. These herbs can be taken as part of a relaxing ritual, such as in a warm herbal tea or mixed with almond or oat milk before bed.

Evening Tea: Add a small amount of ashwagandha powder to warm milk with a dash of honey for a calming bedtime drink.

Sleep-Supportive Tinctures: Use holy basil or ashwagandha tincture to promote relaxation and wind down at night.

Combine with Mindfulness Practices: Stress management is most effective when using a holistic approach. Complement adaptogens with mindfulness practices, such as meditation, deep breathing exercises, or yoga. Adaptogens work at the biochemical level to reduce stress hormones like cortisol, while mindfulness practices help reduce mental stress and improve focus. For instance, taking a small dose of ashwagandha or rhodiola before a meditation session may enhance mental clarity and relaxation, deepening the mindfulness experience.

Stay Hydrated for Better Absorption: Adequate hydration helps with the absorption of many supplements, including adaptogens. Drinking enough water throughout the day ensures that your body can fully utilize the active compounds in these herbs. Aim to drink at least 8 glasses of water daily and consider pairing adaptogens with hydrating foods, like fruits and vegetables, to support absorption and overall wellness.

Personalizing Your Adaptogen Routine

Start with One Adaptogen at a Time: Adaptogens are powerful herbs, so it's wise to introduce them one at a time. Starting with a single adaptogen allows you to observe how it affects your body and to monitor for any side effects. Once you're familiar with its effects, you can gradually introduce additional adaptogens if desired.

Cycle Your Adaptogens: To maintain their effectiveness, consider cycling adaptogens—using them for a few weeks followed by a short break. For instance, you might use ashwagandha daily for 8 weeks, then take a 1-2 week break before resuming. Cycling helps prevent your body from developing a tolerance and ensures sustained benefits over the long term.

Combine Adaptogens for Synergistic Effects: Some adaptogens complement each other when used together. For example, ashwagandha and holy basil both reduce stress and promote relaxation, making them a good pairing for evening use. Rhodiola and maca both support energy and stamina, making them a powerful morning combination for those with busy schedules or high physical demands. Look for combination formulas that are specifically crafted for energy, focus, or stress relief.

Adjust Dosages According to Your Goals: The recommended dosage for each adaptogen varies depending on its intended use. For example, lower doses of rhodiola are better for cognitive function, while higher doses support physical endurance. Similarly, ashwagandha is often taken in smaller doses for relaxation and larger doses for reducing cortisol levels. Consult with a healthcare provider to tailor dosages to your specific needs.

Avoiding Potential Pitfalls and Optimizing Safety

Consult with a Healthcare Professional: Before starting any new supplement, especially if you are on medication or have existing health conditions, consult with a healthcare provider. Some adaptogens, like ginseng, may interact with medications such as blood thinners. A healthcare professional can help you create a safe, effective plan that aligns with your health profile.

Monitor for Side Effects: While adaptogens are generally safe, some people may experience mild side effects like digestive discomfort, headaches, or drowsiness. Monitor how your body reacts, and adjust dosages if necessary. If you experience any adverse effects, discontinue use and consult a healthcare professional.

Keep a Wellness Journal: Tracking your progress can help you understand how adaptogens and lifestyle practices are affecting your energy, stress levels, and overall wellness. A wellness journal can help you record dosages, combinations, and any physical or mental changes you observe. This can provide valuable insights into what works best for you and help you refine your routine over time.

Integrating adaptogenic herbs with a well-rounded lifestyle is a powerful way to enhance energy, resilience to stress, and overall well-being. By selecting high-quality products, incorporating them into a balanced diet, supporting them with exercise, mindfulness, and sleep routines, and consulting healthcare professionals when needed, you can maximize the benefits of these traditional remedies. Adaptogens, paired with modern lifestyle strategies, offer a holistic approach to wellness, helping you build a sustainable routine for a healthier, more balanced life.

Energizing and Revitalizing Recipes: Adaptogenic Beverages, Smoothies, and Snacks to Boost Energy and Overall Well-Being

This collection of 25 recipes is designed to naturally increase energy, stamina, and mental clarity through the use of adaptogenic herbs and other nutrient-rich ingredients. Adaptogens like ginseng, ashwagandha, maca, and rhodiola are combined with fruits, nuts, and superfoods to create delicious beverages, smoothies, and snacks that support physical endurance, reduce stress, and enhance general well-being. Each recipe provides specific dosages of adaptogens, preparation instructions, and suggested variations to suit your unique needs. These recipes can be easily incorporated into a daily routine, helping you stay energized and resilient, whether at work, at the gym, or throughout a busy day.

25 recipes for mental well-being

126. Ginseng & Green Tea Energy Tonic
Description: A refreshing tonic for sustained energy and mental clarity.
Ingredients:
 1 cup brewed **green tea**
 1/2 tsp **ginseng powder** (or 1 ginseng capsule, opened)
 1 tsp **honey** (optional)
Instructions:
 Brew green tea and let it cool slightly.
 Stir in ginseng powder and honey if desired.
Variation:
 Add Lemon: Squeeze in fresh lemon juice for an extra boost of vitamin C.
How to Use: Sip in the morning or early afternoon for an energy lift.

---

127. Maca & Banana Smoothie
Description: A creamy, energizing smoothie to start the day.
Ingredients:
 1 banana
 1/2 tsp **maca powder**
 1 cup **almond milk** (or other milk of choice)
Instructions:
 Blend all ingredients until smooth.
 Serve immediately.
Variation:
 Add Peanut Butter: Add 1 tbsp peanut butter for extra protein.
How to Use: Enjoy as a morning or pre-workout smoothie.

128. Ashwagandha Golden Milk Latte

Description: A warm, comforting drink to reduce stress and promote relaxation.
Ingredients:
- 1 cup **almond milk**
- 1/2 tsp **ashwagandha powder**
- 1/2 tsp **turmeric powder**
- 1 tsp **honey** (optional)

Instructions:
- Heat almond milk and stir in ashwagandha, turmeric, and honey.
- Stir well and enjoy warm.

Variation:
- **Add Cinnamon**: Sprinkle cinnamon for extra warmth and flavor.

How to Use: Drink in the evening to wind down.

---

129. Rhodiola Rosea Iced Tea

Description: A cooling drink for enhanced stamina and stress relief.
Ingredients:
- 1 cup brewed **herbal tea**, cooled
- 1/2 tsp **rhodiola powder**
- 1 tsp **lemon juice**

Instructions:
- Stir rhodiola powder and lemon juice into the cooled tea.
- Serve over ice.

Variation:
- **Add Mint**: Garnish with fresh mint leaves for a refreshing twist.

How to Use: Drink before activities requiring focus or physical endurance.

---

130. Cacao & Maca Energy Bites

Description: Nutty and chocolatey snack bites for a quick energy boost.
Ingredients:
- 1 cup **dates**, pitted
- 1/2 cup **almonds**
- 1 tbsp **cacao powder**
- 1/2 tsp **maca powder**

Instructions:
- Blend all ingredients in a food processor until sticky.
- Roll into small balls and refrigerate.

Variation:
- **Add Coconut Flakes**: Roll bites in coconut for extra texture.

How to Use: Enjoy 1-2 bites as an afternoon snack.

---

131. Matcha & Ginseng Smoothie Bowl

Description: A vibrant smoothie bowl packed with antioxidants and adaptogens.
Ingredients:
- 1/2 tsp **matcha powder**
- 1/2 tsp **ginseng powder**
- 1 cup **coconut milk**
- 1/2 cup **frozen mango**

Instructions:
- Blend ingredients until smooth.
- Pour into a bowl and top with fruit or nuts.

Variation:
- **Add Granola**: Sprinkle granola on top for added crunch.

How to Use: Enjoy as a breakfast or post-workout snack.

132. Chia & Holy Basil Hydrating Drink

Description: A refreshing and hydrating drink with adaptogens and fiber.
Ingredients:
- 1 cup **coconut water**
- 1 tsp **chia seeds**
- 1/2 tsp **holy basil (tulsi) powder**

Instructions:
- Stir chia seeds and tulsi powder into coconut water.
- Let sit for 10 minutes before drinking.

Variation:
- **Add Lime**: Squeeze in fresh lime juice for extra zest.

How to Use: Drink mid-morning or mid-afternoon for hydration and energy.

---

133. Maca & Almond Energy Balls

Description: Small, nutrient-dense bites to fuel your day.
Ingredients:
- 1 cup **almonds**
- 1/2 cup **dates**
- 1 tbsp **maca powder**

Instructions:
- Process all ingredients in a food processor until sticky.
- Roll into small balls and refrigerate.

Variation:
- **Add Cinnamon**: Add 1/4 tsp cinnamon for extra warmth.

How to Use: Enjoy 1-2 balls as a snack.

---

134. Ashwagandha & Lavender Evening Tea

Description: A calming tea to ease stress and promote relaxation.
Ingredients:
- 1 cup hot water
- 1/2 tsp **ashwagandha powder**
- 1/2 tsp dried **lavender flowers**

Instructions:
- Steep ashwagandha and lavender in hot water for 5 minutes.
- Strain and sip slowly.

Variation:
- **Add Honey**: Add a spoonful of honey for sweetness.

How to Use: Enjoy in the evening for relaxation.

---

135. Ginger & Holy Basil Immunity Shot

Description: A spicy shot to boost immunity and energy.
Ingredients:
- 1 inch fresh **ginger**, grated
- 1/2 tsp **holy basil powder**
- 1/4 cup **orange juice**

Instructions:
- Combine all ingredients in a small cup.
- Drink in one shot.

Variation:
- **Add Turmeric**: Add a pinch of turmeric for extra benefits.

How to Use: Take in the morning for an immune and energy boost.

136. Green Apple & Rhodiola Smoothie

Description: A tart smoothie to promote focus and reduce fatigue.
Ingredients:
- 1 green apple, chopped
- 1/2 cup **spinach**
- 1/2 tsp **rhodiola powder**
- 1 cup **coconut water**

Instructions:
Blend all ingredients until smooth.

Variation:
Add Ginger: Add 1/4 tsp grated ginger for extra spice.

How to Use: Drink as a morning or midday refresher.

---

137. Cacao & Maca Mocha Latte

Description: A rich, chocolatey drink with a natural energy boost.
Ingredients:
- 1/2 tsp **maca powder**
- 1 tbsp **cacao powder**
- 1 cup **almond milk**

Instructions:
Warm almond milk and stir in maca and cacao.

Variation:
Add Espresso: Add a shot of espresso for extra energy.

How to Use: Enjoy mid-morning or early afternoon for a lift.

---

138. Berry & Holy Basil Smoothie

Description: A vibrant smoothie packed with antioxidants and adaptogens.
Ingredients:
- 1/2 cup **mixed berries** (fresh or frozen)
- 1/2 tsp **holy basil (tulsi) powder**
- 1 cup **coconut water**

Instructions:
Blend all ingredients until smooth.

Variation:
Add Chia Seeds: Add 1 tsp chia seeds for extra fiber and energy.

How to Use: Drink mid-morning or as an afternoon pick-me-up.

---

139. . Adaptogenic Green Smoothie Bowl

Description: A nourishing smoothie bowl with adaptogens and greens.
Ingredients:
- 1/2 cup **spinach**
- 1/2 **banana**
- 1/2 tsp **ashwagandha powder**
- 1 cup **almond milk**

Instructions:
Blend until smooth, then pour into a bowl.
Top with sliced fruit, nuts, or seeds.

Variation:
Add Hemp Seeds: Sprinkle 1 tbsp hemp seeds for protein.

How to Use: Perfect for a breakfast bowl to start the day.

140. Maca & Cacao Protein Balls

Description: Bite-sized snacks for a boost of energy and focus.
Ingredients:
- 1 cup **oats**
- 1 tbsp **maca powder**
- 1 tbsp **cacao powder**
- 1/4 cup **almond butter**

Instructions:
- Mix all ingredients and roll into balls.
- Refrigerate until firm.

Variation:
- **Add Coconut Flakes**: Roll in coconut flakes for added flavor.

How to Use: Eat 1-2 balls before a workout or during a busy day.

---

141. Ginger & Ginseng Detox Drink

Description: A cleansing drink with a gentle energy boost.
Ingredients:
- 1 inch fresh **ginger**, grated
- 1/2 tsp **ginseng powder**
- 1 cup warm **water**

Instructions:
- Steep ginger in warm water, then stir in ginseng powder.

Variation:
- **Add Lemon**: Squeeze in fresh lemon juice for an added cleanse.

How to Use: Drink first thing in the morning.

---

142. Coconut & Rhodiola Energy Smoothie

Description: A tropical smoothie for mental clarity and vitality.
Ingredients:
- 1/2 cup **pineapple chunks**
- 1/2 cup **coconut milk**
- 1/2 tsp **rhodiola powder**

Instructions:
- Blend ingredients until smooth.

Variation:
- **Add Spinach**: Add a handful of spinach for added greens.

How to Use: Ideal for an energizing breakfast or snack.

---

143. Ashwagandha & Berry Yogurt Parfait

Description: A layered parfait for sustained energy and relaxation.
Ingredients:
- 1/2 cup **Greek yogurt**
- 1/2 tsp **ashwagandha powder**
- 1/4 cup **mixed berries**

Instructions:
- Mix ashwagandha with yogurt.
- Layer with berries in a glass.

Variation:
- **Add Granola**: Sprinkle granola for crunch and fiber.

How to Use: Enjoy as a breakfast or mid-morning snack.

144. Green Tea & Mint Energy Iced Tea

Description: A refreshing, antioxidant-rich iced tea.
Ingredients:
- 1 cup brewed **green tea**, cooled
- 1/2 tsp **rhodiola powder**
- Fresh **mint leaves**

Instructions:
Mix rhodiola powder and green tea, then add mint leaves.

Variation:
Add Lemon Slices: For added flavor and vitamin C.

How to Use: Perfect for a refreshing drink during a busy day.

---

145. Maca & Coconut Almond Butter Cups

Description: Creamy snack cups for an energizing treat.
Ingredients:
- 1/2 cup **almond butter**
- 1/2 tsp **maca powder**
- 1 tbsp **coconut oil**

Instructions:
Melt coconut oil and mix with almond butter and maca.
Pour into small cups and freeze.

Variation:
Add Dark Chocolate Drizzle: Drizzle melted dark chocolate for a touch of sweetness.

How to Use: Enjoy 1-2 cups for an afternoon boost.

---

146. Turmeric & Ashwagandha Warm Lemon Drink

Description: A warm, anti-inflammatory drink to start the day.
Ingredients:
- 1/2 tsp **ashwagandha powder**
- 1/4 tsp **turmeric powder**
- Juice of 1/2 **lemon**

Instructions:
Mix ashwagandha, turmeric, and lemon juice with warm water.

Variation:
Add Honey: Sweeten with honey if desired.

How to Use: Sip in the morning for a gentle wake-up.

---

147. 22. Berry & Maca Recovery Smoothie

Description: A rejuvenating smoothie post-workout.
Ingredients:
- 1/2 cup **mixed berries**
- 1/2 tsp **maca powder**
- 1 cup **almond milk**

Instructions:
Blend ingredients until smooth.

Variation:
Add Protein Powder: For additional post-workout recovery.

How to Use: Drink immediately after exercise.

148. 23. Adaptogenic Overnight Oats

Description: A convenient, energy-boosting breakfast.
Ingredients:
- 1/2 cup **rolled oats**
- 1/2 tsp **ashwagandha powder**
- 1 cup **almond milk**

Instructions:
- Mix oats, ashwagandha, and almond milk in a jar.
- Refrigerate overnight.

Variation:
- **Add Fruit**: Top with fresh berries in the morning.

How to Use: Enjoy as a grab-and-go breakfast.

---

149. 24. Ginseng & Honey Tonic

Description: A warm, revitalizing tonic for a natural energy lift.
Ingredients:
- 1/2 tsp **ginseng powder**
- 1 cup warm **water**
- 1 tsp **honey**

Instructions:
- Mix ginseng powder with water and honey.

Variation:
- **Add Lemon**: Add lemon juice for extra zest.

How to Use: Drink in the morning or mid-afternoon.

---

150. 25. Cacao & Ashwagandha Hot Chocolate

Description: A comforting, stress-relieving hot chocolate.
Ingredients:
- 1 cup **almond milk**
- 1 tbsp **cacao powder**
- 1/2 tsp **ashwagandha powder**

Instructions:
- Warm almond milk and stir in cacao and ashwagandha powder.

Variation:
- **Add Cinnamon**: Add a dash of cinnamon for extra warmth.

How to Use: Enjoy as an evening treat to unwind.

These recipes offer a range of delicious options to incorporate adaptogens and other energy-supportive ingredients into your diet. Each drink, smoothie, and snack can be enjoyed at specific times for optimal energy and well-being, providing a natural way to feel revitalized and resilient throughout the day.

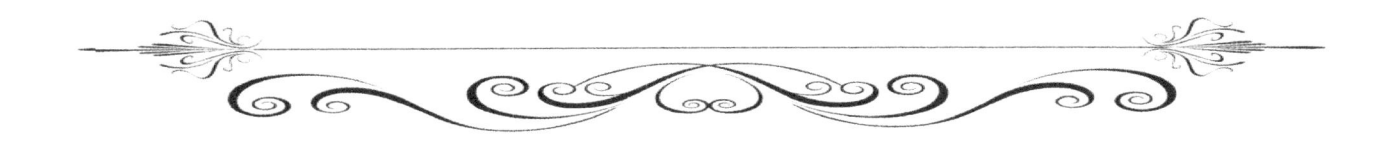

Chapter 8

Myths and Truths about Natural Remedies

Popular Remedies and Science: What Really Works and What Doesn't
Traditional remedies have gained popularity for their natural approach to health, but with the explosion of wellness trends, it can be challenging to know which ones actually work. Scientific studies have shed light on the effectiveness of various popular natural remedies, validating some and debunking others. Here's a closer look at popular remedies, backed by research, to help you understand what works and what doesn't when it comes to natural solutions for health and wellness.

Remedies That Really Work

Garlic for Heart Health

Science Says: Garlic has been extensively studied for its cardiovascular benefits. Research shows that garlic can lower blood pressure, reduce cholesterol levels, and improve overall heart health. The active compound, allicin, has antioxidant and anti-inflammatory properties that support blood vessel health and reduce arterial plaque buildup.

Effective Use: Fresh garlic, garlic oil, or garlic supplements standardized for allicin content are considered effective. Studies recommend around 600-1,200 mg of garlic extract daily.

Ginger for Nausea and Digestive Health

Science Says: Ginger is one of the most well-researched natural remedies, especially for treating nausea and digestive discomfort. Studies have shown ginger's effectiveness in reducing nausea from morning sickness, chemotherapy, and post-surgery recovery. Its compounds, gingerol and shogaol, help relax gastrointestinal muscles and reduce inflammation.

Effective Use: Consuming 1-1.5 grams of fresh or dried ginger per day can reduce nausea. Ginger can be taken as tea, capsules, or chewed raw.

Turmeric for Inflammation

Science Says: Turmeric contains curcumin, a compound with strong anti-inflammatory and antioxidant properties. Numerous studies support turmeric's role in reducing inflammation, which can help manage conditions like arthritis, inflammatory bowel disease, and even heart disease. However, curcumin's low bioavailability has led scientists to pair it with black pepper or fats to enhance absorption.

Effective Use: Studies suggest taking 500-1,000 mg of curcumin with piperine (black pepper extract) daily. Turmeric can be used in cooking, but for therapeutic doses, standardized supplements are recommended.

Peppermint for Irritable Bowel Syndrome (IBS)

Science Says: Research has shown that peppermint oil can help alleviate symptoms of IBS, such as bloating, gas, and abdominal pain. The menthol in peppermint oil has a relaxing effect on the muscles of the gastrointestinal tract, reducing spasms and discomfort.

Effective Use: Enteric-coated peppermint oil capsules (0.2-0.4 mL of peppermint oil per capsule) are typically taken before meals to prevent irritation and provide relief from IBS symptoms.

Ashwagandha for Stress and Anxiety

Science Says: Ashwagandha is a powerful adaptogen shown to lower cortisol levels, reduce anxiety, and improve mental clarity. Several studies have confirmed its effectiveness in reducing stress and anxiety symptoms by supporting adrenal health and modulating the body's response to stress.

Effective Use: The recommended dosage is 300-600 mg of ashwagandha root extract daily. Ashwagandha is commonly consumed as capsules or mixed into warm milk or tea.

Chamomile for Sleep and Relaxation

Science Says: Chamomile has been shown to promote relaxation and improve sleep quality. Studies indicate that the flavonoid apigenin in chamomile binds to receptors in the brain, promoting relaxation and reducing insomnia symptoms.

Effective Use: Chamomile tea (1-2 cups) is a popular and gentle way to enjoy its benefits. Chamomile extract, available in capsules or tinctures, can also be effective.

Remedies That Lack Strong Scientific Evidence

Apple Cider Vinegar for Weight Loss

Science Says: While apple cider vinegar (ACV) has become popular for weight loss, studies on its effectiveness are limited and mixed. Some small studies have suggested that ACV may help reduce appetite or slightly lower blood sugar levels, but the weight loss benefits are not conclusive.

Conclusion: ACV can be used in small amounts (1-2 tablespoons diluted in water) as part of a healthy diet, but it's not a proven weight loss aid. Excessive use may lead to tooth enamel erosion and digestive issues.

Essential Oils for Treating Illnesses

Science Says: Essential oils like lavender, eucalyptus, and tea tree oil are commonly used for relaxation, skincare, and cleaning. While there is some evidence supporting their use for mood enhancement and mild skin issues, there's limited scientific support for claims that they can cure serious health conditions or infections.

Conclusion: Essential oils are best used for aromatherapy, mood support, or skincare, but they should not be relied on as a cure for diseases. Always dilute essential oils and avoid ingesting them unless supervised by a healthcare professional.

Detox Teas and Juice Cleanses

Science Says: The liver and kidneys naturally detoxify the body, so there is limited scientific evidence that detox teas or juice cleanses provide additional benefits. Some detox products may cause short-term weight loss due to their diuretic or laxative effects, but these results are usually temporary.

Conclusion: While juice cleanses can provide nutrients, a balanced diet with plenty of fiber, water, and healthy foods is more effective for long-term health. Detox teas, especially those with laxatives, can lead to dehydration and electrolyte imbalances if used excessively.

Coconut Oil for Heart Health

Science Says: While coconut oil has been touted for its health benefits, its high saturated fat content has raised concerns among experts. Research on coconut oil's effects on heart health is mixed, with some studies suggesting that it raises both LDL (bad) and HDL (good) cholesterol levels.

Conclusion: Coconut oil can be used in moderation as part of a balanced diet, but it's not a miracle food for heart health. Healthier fats, like olive oil, are more beneficial for cardiovascular health.

Collagen Supplements for Skin Health

Science Says: Collagen supplements are marketed for skin health, but the evidence on their effectiveness is limited. While some studies show that collagen may improve skin elasticity slightly, results vary, and the body breaks down collagen into amino acids, so the effects are not direct.

Conclusion: Eating a balanced diet with protein, vitamin C, and other skin-supportive nutrients may be as effective as taking collagen supplements. Collagen's effects on skin health are still under investigation.

Remedies That Show Potential But Need More Research

CBD Oil for Anxiety and Pain Relief

Science Says: Cannabidiol (CBD) has shown potential for reducing anxiety, pain, and inflammation in early studies. However, more research is needed to confirm these effects, and results vary widely depending on dosage and the individual.

Conclusion: CBD oil shows promise as a natural remedy for anxiety and pain, but high-quality studies are still limited. It's best to consult a healthcare provider for guidance on dosage and usage.

Adaptogenic Mushrooms for Immune Support

Science Says: Mushrooms like reishi, lion's mane, and chaga contain compounds that may support immune health and reduce inflammation. While early studies are promising, more research is needed to understand their full effects.

Conclusion: Adaptogenic mushrooms can be included in the diet or taken as supplements for potential immune support, but they should not replace standard treatments for immune health.

Honey for Cough Relief

Science Says: Honey has shown some effectiveness in relieving coughs, particularly in children. Its soothing effect may coat the throat, providing temporary relief. However, honey is not a cure and should not be given to children under one year old.

Conclusion: Honey can be helpful for temporary cough relief, especially when mixed with warm tea, but it's not a replacement for other treatments if symptoms persist.

While many popular natural remedies have strong scientific support, others lack sufficient evidence or require further study to confirm their effectiveness. When exploring natural remedies, it's essential to consider the available research and consult with healthcare providers to ensure safe and effective use. By focusing on well-supported remedies like garlic, ginger, and turmeric, and being cautious with trends that lack strong evidence, you can make informed choices that support long-term health and wellness.

Common Misconceptions: How to Avoid Traps and Myths About Natural Remedies

The world of natural remedies is filled with exciting claims, but it's also rife with misconceptions and myths that can mislead people into using ineffective or even harmful products. While natural remedies offer many potential health benefits, it's essential to approach them with a balanced perspective and an understanding of what the evidence truly supports. Here are some of the most common misconceptions about natural remedies and practical ways to avoid falling into these traps.

"Natural" Means Safe

The Misconception: Many people assume that because a remedy is natural, it's automatically safe and free from side effects.

The Reality: Natural doesn't always mean safe. Just as with conventional medicine, natural remedies can have powerful effects and may interact with medications, cause allergies, or lead to unwanted side effects. For example, while garlic is beneficial for heart health, it can act as a blood thinner and may not be suitable for people on anticoagulant medications. Similarly, some essential oils, such as tea tree oil, can be toxic if ingested and cause skin irritation if used undiluted.

How to Avoid This Trap:
Always research the safety profile of a natural remedy before using it, especially if you have pre-existing health conditions or are taking medications.
Consult a healthcare professional to ensure a remedy is safe for you, particularly when it involves potent herbs, essential oils, or supplements.

More Is Better

The Misconception: If a small dose of a natural remedy works, a larger dose will be even more effective.

The Reality: Many people mistakenly believe that increasing the dose of a natural supplement will enhance its benefits. In reality, higher doses can lead to toxicity or adverse effects. For example, excessive intake of vitamin C can cause digestive issues, and too much fish oil can thin the blood and increase the risk of bleeding. More is not always better; often, a balanced dose is most effective and safest.

How to Avoid This Trap:
Follow recommended dosages provided on product labels or advised by healthcare professionals.
Begin with the lowest effective dose, especially if it's your first time trying a remedy, to gauge your body's reaction before increasing the amount.

Natural Remedies Work Instantly

The Misconception: Natural remedies provide quick results, just like some over-the-counter or prescription medications.

The Reality: Unlike pharmaceuticals that often act quickly, natural remedies usually work gradually and may require consistent use over weeks or even months to show noticeable effects. For example, adaptogens like ashwagandha and rhodiola take time to balance stress hormones and build resilience to stress, and turmeric may need several weeks to reduce inflammation.

How to Avoid This Trap:
Have realistic expectations and allow time for natural remedies to work, as they often address the root cause of issues rather than just alleviating symptoms.
Consistency is key. Regular, daily use often provides better results than using a remedy sporadically.

All Health Claims Are Created Equal

**The Misconcepti
on:** Every health claim about natural remedies is supported by solid evidence.

The Reality: While many health claims for natural remedies are based on tradition and anecdotal reports, they aren't always backed by rigorous scientific studies. For example, while apple cider vinegar is promoted for weight loss, the scientific support for this claim is limited and mixed. Similarly, while some people use coconut oil for heart health, its high saturated fat content makes its cardiovascular benefits questionable.

How to Avoid This Trap:
Seek out reputable sources and check for scientific evidence supporting a remedy's claims. Look for studies published in peer-reviewed journals.
Be cautious of exaggerated or "miracle cure" claims, especially if they seem too good to be true. Reliable products tend to provide honest, science-backed claims without sensationalism.

Traditional Use Equals Scientific Validation

The Misconception: If a natural remedy has been used for centuries, it must be scientifically effective.

The Reality: While traditional use can provide valuable insights, it doesn't guarantee scientific effectiveness. Many traditional remedies are indeed beneficial and supported by research, such as ginger for nausea and turmeric for inflammation. However, others lack robust evidence, and traditional use alone is not always a substitute for scientific validation.

How to Avoid This Trap:
Use traditional remedies as a starting point, but look for modern research to confirm their efficacy and safety.
Be aware that the strength, purity, and preparation methods may differ between traditional and modern uses, affecting their potency and safety.

If It's a Popular Trend, It Must Work

The Misconception: Remedies trending in wellness circles, such as detox teas, juice cleanses, or charcoal supplements, must be effective.

The Reality: Just because a remedy is popular doesn't mean it's effective or necessary. Detox teas, for instance, may provide temporary weight loss due to their laxative effects, but they don't genuinely "detoxify" the body, as the liver and kidneys are naturally responsible for detoxification. Similarly, charcoal supplements can interfere with nutrient absorption and are not advisable unless recommended by a healthcare provider for specific cases.

How to Avoid This Trap:
Approach trends with a healthy dose of skepticism. Just because a remedy is widely marketed or endorsed by influencers doesn't mean it's beneficial.
Focus on building a balanced lifestyle with proven wellness practices—such as a nutritious diet, regular exercise, and stress management—rather than relying on trends.

"All-Natural" Means It's Free of Harmful Ingredients

The Misconception: Products labeled as "all-natural" are pure and don't contain any harmful ingredients.

The Reality: The term "natural" is not strictly regulated and can be misleading. A product labeled "natural" might still contain artificial additives, preservatives, or allergens.

Additionally, certain natural substances, like heavy metals or contaminants, can occasionally be present in herbal products or supplements.

How to Avoid This Trap:
Always read ingredient lists carefully, even on products labeled as natural.
Choose brands that offer transparency in sourcing, manufacturing, and testing, and look for certifications like organic, third-party testing, or non-GMO.

One Remedy Works for Everyone

The Misconception: If a remedy works well for one person, it will work for everyone.

The Reality: Everyone's body reacts differently to natural remedies due to unique genetics, health conditions, and lifestyle factors. For instance, adaptogens like rhodiola may provide energy for some people but could cause drowsiness in others. Similarly, certain herbs like valerian root may aid sleep for some individuals but cause vivid dreams or restlessness for others.

How to Avoid This Trap:
Start with a small dose and monitor how your body responds before increasing the dosage or committing to regular use.
Pay attention to your unique health needs and consult a healthcare provider if you're unsure about trying a new remedy.

Natural Remedies Don't Interact with Medications

The Misconception: Because they're natural, these remedies won't interfere with prescription medications.

The Reality: Natural remedies can interact with medications, either enhancing or diminishing their effects. For example, St. John's Wort can interfere with antidepressants, while ginkgo biloba can increase bleeding risk when taken with blood thinners. Ignoring these interactions can lead to dangerous side effects or decreased effectiveness of prescribed treatments.

How to Avoid This Trap:
Always disclose any natural supplements or remedies you're taking to your healthcare provider.
Avoid combining natural remedies with medications unless you have confirmed they are safe to use together.

Natural Remedies Are a Substitute for Medical Treatment

The Misconception: Natural remedies can replace conventional medical treatments for serious health conditions.

The Reality: While natural remedies can complement medical treatments, they are not a substitute for professional healthcare, particularly in the case of serious conditions like cancer, heart disease, or severe mental health disorders. Self-treating with natural remedies in place of proven medical interventions can delay essential care and lead to worsening health outcomes.

How to Avoid This Trap:
Use natural remedies as a supplement to, rather than a replacement for, medical treatment. Work closely with your healthcare provider to determine a balanced approach that combines both natural and conventional treatments if appropriate.
Natural remedies can offer powerful benefits for health and well-being, but understanding their true effects requires discernment and a scientific approach. By avoiding common misconceptions—such as "natural means safe" or "more is better"—and focusing on evidence-based use, you can make the most of these remedies without falling into the traps of myths and exaggerated claims. Informed use of natural remedies, alongside professional guidance and healthy lifestyle habits, provides a balanced and safe path to wellness.

Verifying Sources and Products: Tips for Identifying Safe and Reliable Products

With the wide array of natural health products on the market, it's crucial to identify those that are both safe and effective. The quality and reliability of a product depend on its sourcing, manufacturing practices, ingredient purity, and transparency in labeling. Verifying sources and choosing high-quality products can help you make informed decisions and avoid ineffective or potentially harmful items. Here are practical tips on how to ensure that the products you select are trustworthy and meet high standards.

Look for Third-Party Testing and Certifications

What to Look For:
Reputable supplements and natural health products often display third-party certifications or testing labels on their packaging. These labels indicate that an independent organization has verified the product for quality, potency, and purity.
Common third-party testing organizations include **USP (United States Pharmacopeia), NSF International, ConsumerLab**, and **Informed Choice**.

Why It Matters:
Third-party testing ensures that the product contains the ingredients listed on the label in the stated amounts and is free from harmful contaminants like heavy metals, pesticides, and microbes.

These certifications offer peace of mind, knowing that the product has passed rigorous quality standards.

How to Use This Tip:
Check the packaging or product website for certification seals.
Verify that the certification organization is credible and widely recognized.

Choose Products from Transparent, Reputable Brands

What to Look For:
Reputable companies are transparent about their manufacturing processes, ingredient sourcing, and quality control measures. They often provide detailed information about these practices on their websites or packaging.
Look for brands that use **Good Manufacturing Practices (GMP)**, which follow FDA-approved guidelines for quality and safety in production.

Why It Matters:
Transparency about sourcing, ingredient quality, and manufacturing practices reflects a company's commitment to quality and customer safety. Reliable brands are upfront about their practices and adhere to strict standards.

How to Use This Tip:
Visit the company's website and look for information about sourcing, manufacturing, and quality control.
Be cautious if this information is absent or if the company uses vague language.

Review the Ingredients and Avoid Unnecessary Additives

What to Look For:
High-quality products generally have simple, straightforward ingredient lists. Avoid products with artificial colors, flavors, preservatives, or fillers, as these are often unnecessary and can cause allergic reactions or other health issues.
Be especially wary of products containing vague ingredients such as "proprietary blend" without specifying the exact amounts, as this can obscure how much of each ingredient you are actually consuming.

Why It Matters:
Minimal additives reduce the risk of adverse reactions and ensure that you are getting pure, concentrated ingredients.
Transparent ingredient lists allow you to verify that each component has a purpose and isn't included just to bulk up the product.

How to Use This Tip:
Read the label carefully, and if the ingredient list is long or contains unfamiliar terms, do some research on each ingredient.
Opt for products that provide clear information on active ingredients and avoid those with generic terms like "proprietary blend."

Research the Manufacturer's Reputation and Track Record

What to Look For:
Established brands with a strong reputation often have a long-standing track record of producing quality products. Check if the brand has positive reviews from verified purchasers and any endorsements from health professionals or reputable organizations.
Look out for any recalls or quality issues reported in the past, as well as any FDA warnings or lawsuits.

Why It Matters:
A brand's history in the market and consumer feedback can indicate reliability and trustworthiness. Brands with numerous recalls or legal issues may have quality control problems that impact product safety.

How to Use This Tip:
Read customer reviews on verified platforms, such as the brand's website, online retailers, or independent review sites.
Use websites like the **FDA** or **Better Business Bureau (BBB)** to check for any recalls, warnings, or unresolved consumer complaints.

Understand the Dosage and Potency of Ingredients

What to Look For:
High-quality products provide clear information on dosages for each ingredient, allowing you to determine if the dosage aligns with research-based recommendations.
Be cautious of supplements with "proprietary blends," which may not specify how much of each ingredient is included, potentially leading to subtherapeutic doses or unwanted side effects.

Why It Matters:
Understanding dosages helps you select products that are both safe and effective. Knowing the potency of each ingredient ensures you are taking the appropriate amount for desired effects without risking overuse.

How to Use This Tip:
Look for clear labeling that specifies the exact dosage of each active ingredient.
Cross-check recommended dosages with credible sources to ensure they are within safe and effective ranges.

Verify Product Claims with Scientific Evidence

What to Look For:
Reputable companies base their product claims on research, often citing studies or scientific evidence to back up their products' benefits. Look for claims supported by real research, rather than vague promises like "miracle cure" or "guaranteed results."
Check if the company's website includes links to peer-reviewed studies or research summaries.

Why It Matters:
Verified scientific claims help ensure the product's efficacy and align with realistic health outcomes. Misleading claims can lead to disappointment and potential misuse of the product.

How to Use This Tip:
Search for credible studies supporting the product's claims and review scientific literature if available.
Avoid products that make exaggerated or unrealistic promises, as these are often red flags.

Be Wary of Products That Are "Too Good to Be True"

What to Look For:
Products promising quick results, miracle cures, or "no side effects" are often marketing gimmicks. Genuine health supplements and remedies typically require consistent use and may not work for everyone in the same way.
Watch out for phrases like "guaranteed cure," "overnight results," or "all-natural miracle."

Why It Matters:
Misleading claims can create false expectations, leading to disappointment or improper use. Reliable products tend to provide honest claims about what they can and cannot do.

How to Use This Tip:
Approach "miracle" products with caution and skepticism, as legitimate products rarely promise immediate results or cures.
Check if the company's language aligns with realistic expectations based on scientific research.

Consult a Healthcare Professional When in Doubt

What to Look For:
For any questions about the safety, dosage, or interactions of a product, seek advice from a healthcare professional who is knowledgeable about supplements. They can provide insights based on your personal health history and needs.

Why It Matters:
Professional guidance helps you make safe and informed decisions, especially when introducing a new product that could potentially interact with medications or pre-existing conditions.

How to Use This Tip:
Reach out to your doctor, pharmacist, or a certified dietitian before starting any new supplement or natural remedy, especially if you are on medication or have a chronic health condition.

Buy from Trusted Sources and Retailers

What to Look For:
Purchase products from reputable sources, such as established health food stores, certified online retailers, or directly from the manufacturer's website. Be cautious with products sold on online marketplaces where counterfeit or expired products may be listed.

Why It Matters:
Purchasing from trusted sources reduces the risk of receiving counterfeit, expired, or substandard products. Reputable retailers also offer customer service and return policies if the product does not meet expectations.

How to Use This Tip:
Avoid buying from unknown or unverified sellers, especially if the price seems too low compared to other sources.
Check if the retailer has a good reputation for authenticity and quality.

Track Your Experience and Results

What to Look For:
Once you start using a product, monitor your body's response, noting any positive effects, side effects, or lack of noticeable results. Tracking your experience allows you to evaluate the product's effectiveness and make informed decisions about continued use.

Why It Matters:
Tracking your experience helps you determine if the product is meeting your expectations and if any adjustments are needed. It also provides valuable information should you need to discuss the product with a healthcare provider.

How to Use This Tip:
Keep a journal or use a tracking app to record your daily intake, dosage, and any effects you notice.
Periodically review your notes to assess whether the product is benefiting your health goals.
 Identifying safe and reliable products in the natural health market requires careful evaluation and a commitment to quality. By verifying third-party testing, researching the manufacturer, reading ingredient lists, and being cautious with product claims, you can confidently choose products that are effective and safe for your health needs. Combining these practices with professional guidance and personal tracking empowers you to make informed choices that support long-term wellness and well-being.

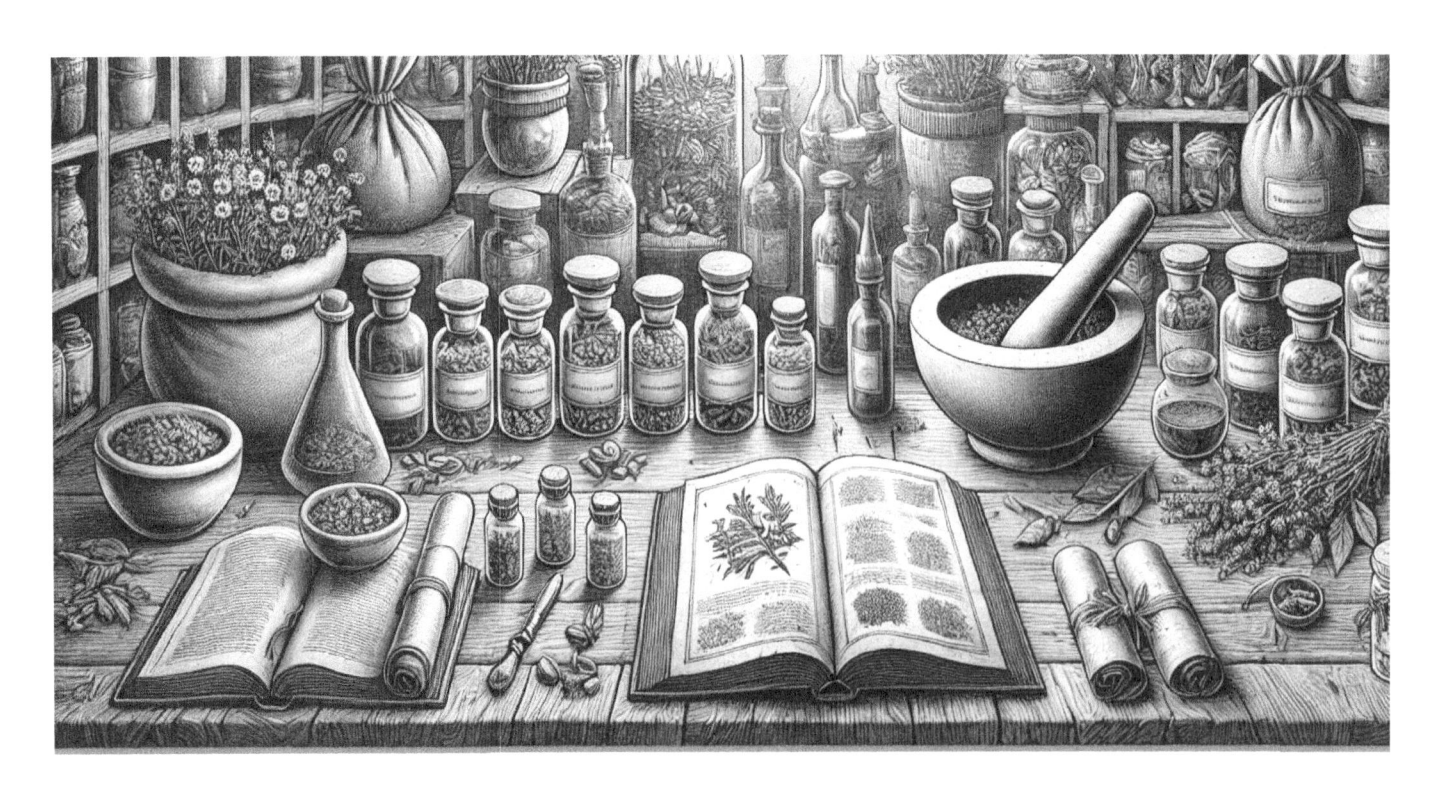

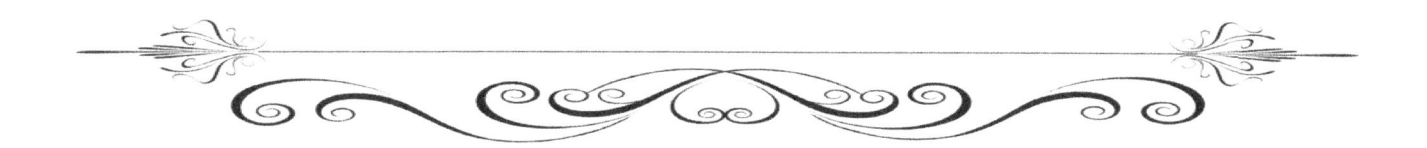

Chapter 9

Guidelines for Safe Use

Principles for Safe and Mindful Use: How and When to Combine Natural Remedies and Medications

As interest in natural remedies grows, more people are looking to integrate these solutions alongside conventional medications. While natural remedies can complement traditional treatments, they must be combined thoughtfully to ensure safety and effectiveness. Certain herbs, supplements, and essential oils may interact with medications, either enhancing or inhibiting their effects, which can lead to unintended consequences. Here are key principles to help guide the safe and informed use of natural remedies alongside medications.

Understand Potential Interactions

Why It Matters:
Many natural remedies contain active compounds that can interact with medications in ways similar to pharmaceuticals. For example, St. John's Wort is a natural herb used for mood support, but it can interfere with the effectiveness of antidepressants and increase the risk of side effects. Similarly, ginkgo biloba may increase bleeding risks when taken with blood-thinning medications.

How to Approach It:
Research potential interactions between any natural remedy and the medications you're taking. Reliable resources include databases like the **National Institutes of Health (NIH)**, **MedlinePlus**, and **Natural Medicines**.
Keep in mind that interactions can vary depending on the dose and frequency of the remedy.

Consult Your Healthcare Provider

Why It Matters:
Medical professionals, especially those familiar with integrative medicine, can provide personalized advice based on your health profile, current medications, and goals for using natural remedies. They can help you understand which remedies are safe to combine with your medications and which should be avoided.

How to Approach It:
When starting a new natural remedy, discuss it with your doctor or pharmacist to identify any potential interactions or side effects.
Inform your healthcare provider about all the natural supplements, herbs, and over-the-counter products you're taking so they can help create a safe plan for combining them with medications.

Start Low and Go Slow

Why It Matters:
When introducing a new natural remedy alongside a medication, starting with a low dose allows you to observe how your body responds. This cautious approach helps minimize the risk of interactions and side effects.

How to Approach It:
Begin with a small dose of the natural remedy, especially if it's your first time trying it, and gradually increase only if no adverse reactions occur.
Keep a close eye on any changes in your body, such as new symptoms or changes in medication efficacy, and report these to your healthcare provider.

Avoid "Stacking" Remedies with Similar Effects
Why It Matters:
Combining remedies and medications that have similar effects can amplify their impact, sometimes leading to unintended consequences. For example, combining multiple sedative herbs, such as valerian and kava, with a prescription sleep aid could lead to excessive drowsiness or respiratory depression.

How to Approach It:
Avoid taking multiple natural remedies or medications that produce the same effect, such as combining several calming herbs with anti-anxiety medications.
Be mindful of combining blood-thinning natural remedies (like garlic, ginkgo, or fish oil) with anticoagulant medications to avoid increased bleeding risk.

Time Dosing Carefully

Why It Matters:
Taking natural remedies and medications at the same time can sometimes lead to competition for absorption or amplify effects unintentionally. For instance, calcium supplements can interfere with the absorption of certain antibiotics if taken simultaneously.

How to Approach It:
Space out natural remedies and medications by a few hours to allow each one to be absorbed independently.
Follow any specific timing recommendations from your healthcare provider, such as taking remedies with meals to aid absorption or before bed for a relaxing effect.

Stick to Recommended Dosages

Why It Matters:
Higher doses of natural remedies don't necessarily mean better results and can increase the risk of interactions or side effects. For example, excessive fish oil intake can thin the blood too much, increasing bleeding risks, especially when combined with blood-thinning medications.

How to Approach It:
Adhere to the recommended dosage provided by your healthcare provider or as indicated on the product label.
Be cautious with high-potency or "concentrated" products, as these may deliver a much higher dose than you would typically get from a natural source.

Monitor for Side Effects and Adjust as Needed

Why It Matters:
Both medications and natural remedies can cause side effects, and combining them can lead to unexpected reactions. Monitoring your health closely when introducing a new remedy helps catch any negative effects early.

How to Approach It:
Keep a health journal to track how you feel after introducing a new remedy or combination. Note any symptoms like headaches, digestive issues, dizziness, or changes in the effectiveness of your medication.
If you notice any side effects or unusual symptoms, discontinue the remedy and consult your healthcare provider.

Choose Reputable Sources and High-Quality Products
Why It Matters:
Poor-quality natural products may contain contaminants or inconsistent amounts of active ingredients, which can increase the risk of interactions. Quality control in supplements is essential to ensure you're consuming safe and effective dosages.
How to Approach It:

Select products from reputable brands that use third-party testing and certification. Look for labels like **USP Verified**, **NSF Certified**, or **ConsumerLab Approved**.
Avoid products with vague ingredient lists, unknown additives, or unclear dosages, especially when you plan to combine them with medications.

Consider Cycling or "Taking Breaks"

Why It Matters:
Taking certain natural remedies long-term may lead to tolerance, reduced effectiveness, or even negative side effects over time. Cycling, or taking breaks from specific remedies, can help maintain their efficacy and reduce potential interactions with medications.

How to Approach It:
Use adaptogens like ashwagandha or ginseng for a few weeks, then take a break before resuming. This approach can help avoid overuse and maintain effectiveness.
Follow your healthcare provider's advice on when and how to cycle specific remedies.

Know When to Avoid Combining Remedies and Medications

Why It Matters:
Certain medications are highly sensitive to interactions, and combining them with natural remedies can pose significant risks. For example, immunosuppressive drugs and certain cancer treatments should not be combined with immune-boosting herbs.

How to Approach It:
Avoid using immune-stimulating remedies (like echinacea) if you're taking immunosuppressants, as they may counteract the medication.
Always double-check with your healthcare provider before combining any remedy with critical or life-sustaining medications, such as anticoagulants, immunosuppressants, or chemotherapy drugs.

Use Natural Remedies to Complement, Not Replace, Medications

Why It Matters:
Natural remedies can support certain health goals, but they are not substitutes for prescribed medications, especially for chronic or serious conditions. Attempting to replace medication with a natural remedy without medical guidance can lead to worsening symptoms or complications.

How to Approach It:
View natural remedies as supportive tools that can enhance well-being or alleviate minor symptoms, rather than as replacements for medications prescribed by a doctor.
Always consult your healthcare provider if you're considering reducing or discontinuing a medication, as they can help you create a safe plan.

Seek Professional Guidance with Complex Health Conditions

Why It Matters:
For complex conditions such as autoimmune disorders, heart disease, or mental health issues, combining remedies and medications can have varied, often unpredictable effects. Professional
guidance is essential in these cases to avoid adverse interactions and achieve a balanced approach to health.

How to Approach It:
Work with an integrative medicine practitioner or a healthcare provider with knowledge in natural therapies who can offer tailored guidance on safe combinations for your specific condition.
In complex cases, prioritize regular check-ins with your healthcare provider to adjust treatments as needed based on your response.
Combining natural remedies with medications requires a mindful, informed approach to ensure safety and maximize benefits. By understanding potential interactions, consulting healthcare providers, sticking to recommended dosages, and monitoring for side effects, you can create a balanced plan that incorporates both traditional and natural therapies. Embracing these principles for safe and conscious use allows you to enjoy the best of both worlds in a way that supports your health and well-being responsibly.

Warnings and Contraindications: Identifying Dangerous Interactions and Recognizing When to Consult a Doctor

While natural remedies can offer valuable support for health and wellness, it's important to be aware of potential dangers when combining them with certain medications or health conditions. Understanding the risks, knowing which interactions to avoid, and recognizing when to seek medical advice can help prevent adverse effects and support safe, effective use. Here's a guide to navigating the complexities of interactions and when to consult a healthcare provider for guidance.

Be Aware of Herb-Drug Interactions

Why It Matters:
Herbs and medications may interact in ways that alter their effects, leading to either amplified or diminished results. For instance, St. John's Wort, commonly used for mild depression, can reduce the effectiveness of certain antidepressants, birth control pills, and blood thinners by increasing the liver's ability to metabolize these drugs.

Examples of Common Herb-Drug Interactions:
St. John's Wort: Interacts with antidepressants, birth control, immunosuppressants, and blood thinners.

Ginkgo Biloba: Increases the risk of bleeding when combined with anticoagulants like warfarin or aspirin.

Garlic: Also a blood thinner, it can increase bleeding risks when taken with anticoagulants.

Ginseng: May interfere with blood pressure medications and blood thinners.

Valerian Root: Has sedative properties that can increase drowsiness when taken with anti-anxiety medications or sleep aids.

How to Approach It:
Before taking any herbal supplement, research potential interactions with your medications and consult a healthcare provider if you're unsure.
Avoid combining multiple supplements or herbs with similar effects (e.g., blood-thinning herbs with anticoagulant drugs) unless advised by a medical professional.

Recognize Conditions that May Be Worsened by Natural Remedies

Why It Matters:
Certain health conditions can be negatively affected by specific natural remedies, even if the remedies are safe for the general population. For example, people with autoimmune diseases are often advised to avoid immune-boosting herbs like echinacea, as these can exacerbate symptoms by stimulating immune activity.

Conditions and Natural Remedies to Be Cautious With:
Autoimmune Diseases: Avoid immune-stimulants like echinacea, ashwagandha, and elderberry, which may worsen symptoms.

Blood Pressure Issues: Licorice root can raise blood pressure and should be avoided by those with hypertension.

Liver Conditions: High doses of green tea extract or kava can stress the liver and should be avoided by people with liver disease.

Kidney Disease: Avoid high doses of certain minerals (like potassium and magnesium supplements) without supervision, as these can exacerbate kidney conditions.

How to Approach It:
If you have a chronic condition, consult your doctor before starting a new remedy to ensure it's safe and appropriate for your situation.
Seek out specific research or guidance on whether the remedy is contraindicated for your condition.

Be Cautious with Remedies That Affect Blood Clotting

Why It Matters:
Many natural remedies, such as garlic, ginkgo biloba, and fish oil, have blood-thinning effects, which can increase the risk of bleeding when taken with anticoagulant medications or before surgical procedures. This effect can be serious, particularly for those who are already on blood-thinning medications like warfarin, aspirin, or clopidogrel.

How to Approach It:
Avoid combining multiple blood-thinning remedies unless approved by your healthcare provider.
If you are scheduled for surgery, discontinue any blood-thinning supplements at least two weeks before your procedure to reduce the risk of excessive bleeding.
Consult your doctor about any supplements that could interfere with blood clotting, especially if you're taking prescription anticoagulants.

Watch for Central Nervous System Interactions

Why It Matters:
Some natural remedies can increase sedation or drowsiness when combined with medications that affect the central nervous system (CNS), such as anti-anxiety drugs, sleep aids, or certain antidepressants. Herbs like valerian root, kava, and passionflower, which have calming effects, can amplify the sedative impact of these medications, potentially leading to excessive drowsiness or respiratory depression.

How to Approach It:
Avoid combining CNS depressant herbs with sedative medications or alcohol unless advised by a healthcare provider.
If you're taking any prescription medication for sleep, anxiety, or mood, consult your doctor before introducing calming herbs to avoid additive effects.

Know When Natural Remedies May Impact Hormone Levels

Why It Matters:
Some herbs and natural supplements can influence hormone levels, which may interfere with hormone-based treatments or conditions. For instance, black cohosh and dong quai, commonly used for menopausal symptoms, can mimic estrogen and may not be suitable for those with estrogen-sensitive conditions, such as certain types of breast cancer.

How to Approach It:
If you are on hormone replacement therapy or have a hormone-sensitive condition, consult your healthcare provider before using herbal supplements that affect hormone levels.
Avoid herbs known to impact hormones, such as maca or saw palmetto, unless advised by a professional.

Avoid Supplements with Undefined Ingredients or "Proprietary Blends"

Why It Matters:
Products labeled as "proprietary blends" often do not disclose exact ingredient amounts, making it difficult to gauge potential interactions or side effects. In addition, products with "natural ingredients" that aren't specified can sometimes include allergens or harmful contaminants.

How to Approach It:
Opt for products with clear labeling that lists all ingredients and dosages.
Avoid supplements with vague ingredient lists or unclear formulations, particularly if you are taking medications that may interact.

Recognize When Symptoms Worsen and Seek Help Immediately

Why It Matters:
Even natural remedies can cause adverse effects, especially when combined with medications. If you notice symptoms like dizziness, nausea, headaches, irregular heartbeat, or difficulty breathing after taking a supplement, it may indicate a dangerous interaction or overdose.

How to Approach It:
Discontinue the remedy immediately and seek medical help if symptoms are severe or persist. Report any side effects to your healthcare provider to help determine the cause and avoid future interactions.

Be Cautious with "Detox" or "Cleansing" Supplements

Why It Matters:
Detox supplements may contain diuretics, laxatives, or high doses of vitamins that can interact with medications or cause dehydration. Detox products are often marketed as safe for everyone, but they can be risky for people with conditions like diabetes, heart disease, or kidney problems.

How to Approach It:
Avoid detox supplements that contain diuretics or laxatives, as they can lead to electrolyte imbalances or dehydration.
Consult your doctor before starting any detox regimen, especially if you are on medications that affect fluid balance or kidney function.

Know When to Consult a Healthcare Provider

When to Seek Professional Advice:

When Starting a New Medication: If you're taking natural supplements and begin a new prescription medication, consult your healthcare provider to identify any potential interactions.

When Adding a New Supplement: Before starting any new herbal supplement, particularly if you're already on medication, check with a medical professional to ensure safety.
Before Surgery or Medical Procedures: Disclose all supplements to your surgeon or doctor before any surgical procedure, as some may increase bleeding risk or interfere with anesthesia.
If You Have a Chronic Condition: Chronic conditions like diabetes, heart disease, liver or kidney disease, and autoimmune disorders can make certain natural remedies unsafe. Consult your healthcare provider before introducing new supplements.
If You Experience Unusual Symptoms: If you notice new or worsening symptoms after taking a supplement, seek immediate medical advice to determine the cause and adjust your regimen as necessary.

Be Open with Your Healthcare Team

Why It Matters:
Many people do not disclose their use of natural supplements to their healthcare providers, but full transparency is crucial for safe, effective treatment. This allows your healthcare provider to make fully informed decisions about your care and help you avoid potential risks.

How to Approach It:
Bring a list of all supplements, herbs, and over-the-counter products you use to your medical appointments.
Update your healthcare team about any changes in your supplement routine, especially if you are managing chronic conditions or undergoing medical treatments.

Safe and effective use of natural remedies requires a thoughtful approach to avoid potentially harmful interactions with medications and to recognize when medical guidance is necessary. By understanding common interactions, being aware of contraindications, and consulting with healthcare providers, you can integrate natural and conventional treatments in a way that prioritizes your health and safety.

Practical Tips and Common Questions: Helpful Advice for Adopting an Integrated and Responsible Approach

Integrating natural remedies with conventional treatments can be an empowering way to support overall health, but it also requires mindful planning, reliable information, and a proactive approach to safety. Here are practical tips and answers to common questions to help you adopt a balanced and responsible approach to using natural remedies alongside traditional medicine, maximizing benefits while minimizing risks.

Start with Clear Health Goals

Why It Matters:
Having clear health goals will help you determine which natural remedies align best with your needs and how they can complement conventional treatments. For example, if your goal is to reduce stress, you might explore adaptogens like ashwagandha or relaxation practices such as mindfulness and meditation.

How to Implement This Tip:
Write down your health goals and prioritize them. Decide what you'd like to improve, whether it's sleep quality, immunity, or energy levels.
Research natural remedies that support your goals and discuss them with a healthcare provider to find the safest and most effective options.

Build a Daily Routine for Consistency

Why It Matters:
Natural remedies often work best when used consistently over time, as many take a few weeks to show effects. A routine ensures you remember to take your supplements and practice self-care.

How to Implement This Tip:
Set a specific time each day to take your supplements, such as with breakfast or before bed, to make it part of your routine.
Use tools like reminder apps, weekly pill organizers, or a health journal to track your daily intake and observe any changes in your well-being.

Start with One Remedy at a Time

Why It Matters:
Adding multiple new remedies at once makes it difficult to know which one is producing specific effects, both positive and negative. Starting with one remedy allows you to gauge its individual impact on your body.

How to Implement This Tip:
Begin with a single remedy and use it consistently for several weeks before adding another.
Track your experience with each remedy, noting any benefits or side effects, and adjust as needed.

Use Reliable Sources for Research

Why It Matters:
There's a vast amount of information online, and not all of it is accurate or backed by science. Using reliable resources ensures that the information you're getting about natural remedies is accurate, safe, and effective.

Where to Look for Reliable Information:
Trusted medical sources, such as the **National Institutes of Health (NIH)**, **World Health Organization (WHO)**, and **Mayo Clinic**, provide evidence-based information on natural remedies.
For supplement specifics, databases like **Natural Medicines** and **MedlinePlus** are valuable for checking interactions, benefits, and recommended dosages.

Keep an Open Dialogue with Your Healthcare Provider

Why It Matters:
Many people don't inform their doctors about the natural supplements they're using, which can lead to missed opportunities for safe integration and potential risks. Open communication allows your healthcare provider to make fully informed recommendations.

How to Implement This Tip:
Bring a complete list of supplements, herbs, and over-the-counter products you're using to each medical appointment. This helps your provider understand your overall health regimen. Update your doctor if you make changes to your routine, such as adding a new remedy or adjusting dosages.

Be Mindful of Possible Side Effects and Interactions

Why It Matters:
Even though natural remedies are often perceived as safe, they can have side effects, especially when combined with medications. Awareness of these potential effects will help you spot any issues early.

How to Implement This Tip:
Research each remedy's potential side effects and interactions, especially if you are taking prescription medications. Resources like MedlinePlus and the NIH's Dietary Supplement Fact Sheets can help.
Keep a journal to track any side effects, and be prepared to discontinue a supplement if it causes discomfort or adverse effects.

Plan Around Your Medications

Why It Matters:
Some natural remedies may compete with medications for absorption or amplify effects, leading to either reduced efficacy or increased side effects. Careful timing of doses can help avoid these interactions.

How to Implement This Tip:
Separate the timing of your medications and natural supplements by a few hours to allow each to be absorbed without interference. For example, calcium can interfere with thyroid medications, so they should be taken at different times.
Consult your doctor or pharmacist on the best timing for each supplement and medication you're using.

Understand When It's Best to Avoid Certain Remedies

Why It Matters:
Certain natural remedies are not suitable for everyone and can pose risks to individuals with specific health conditions. For example, immune-stimulating herbs like echinacea may not be safe for those with autoimmune disorders.

How to Implement This Tip:
Know your health conditions and understand how they may affect your use of natural remedies. Seek professional advice if you're unsure whether a remedy is suitable for you.
Be cautious with remedies that affect blood clotting, hormone levels, or the central nervous system, especially if you're on related medications.

Common Questions About Combining Natural Remedies and Medications

Q: Can I stop taking my medication if a natural remedy seems to work?
Answer: No. Natural remedies are not substitutes for prescribed medications, especially for serious or chronic conditions. Always consult your healthcare provider before making changes to your medication.

Q: Are all "natural" supplements safe to take daily?
Answer: Not all natural supplements are meant for daily use, and some should be cycled. For instance, adaptogens like ashwagandha may be more effective with breaks in between cycles. Check recommendations for each remedy and follow your doctor's advice.

Q: Can natural remedies have side effects if I exceed the dosage?
Answer: Yes. Higher doses can increase the risk of side effects. Always stick to the recommended dose, as "more" is not always "better" and can be dangerous.

Q: How long does it take for natural remedies to work?
Answer: This varies by remedy and individual. Some remedies, like ginger for nausea, act quickly, while others, like adaptogens, may require several weeks of consistent use to show effects.

Q: Should I take a break from supplements if I don't feel any changes?
Answer: Yes, taking a break can be beneficial. It allows you to reassess your health goals and determine if the remedy is effective. Some people cycle certain supplements to prevent tolerance.

Use Technology to Support Your Routine

Why It Matters:
With many remedies to track, technology can help manage your routine, monitor interactions, and even remind you to take supplements.

How to Implement This Tip:
Use health-tracking apps to log your supplement intake and any symptoms. Apps like MyFitnessPal, Cronometer, or customized medication reminders can help keep your routine on track.
Schedule alerts to remind you of dosage timing, especially if spacing out medications and supplements is necessary.

Be Patient and Flexible with Your Health Journey

Why It Matters:
Natural remedies often require time to work and may not show immediate results. Flexibility and patience allow you to observe real changes and make informed adjustments over time.

How to Implement This Tip:
Set realistic expectations and give each remedy time to work. Many natural remedies, like turmeric or ashwagandha, take weeks to build up their effects.
Periodically review your health goals, and be open to adjusting your routine based on what you find most effective and enjoyable.

Trust Your Body and Seek Guidance When Needed

Why It Matters:
Being attuned to your body's responses is essential for recognizing which remedies work best for you. Sometimes, side effects or new symptoms may indicate a need for professional advice.

How to Implement This Tip:
Listen to your body's feedback, and discontinue any remedy that causes discomfort or negative effects.
Don't hesitate to reach out to your healthcare provider for guidance, especially when managing new or complex health conditions.

Adopting an integrated, responsible approach to combining natural remedies and conventional treatments can support your overall wellness journey. By setting clear goals, consulting trusted sources, and maintaining open communication with healthcare professionals, you can enjoy the benefits of natural remedies while staying mindful of potential risks. With patience, consistency, and regular assessments, a balanced approach can enhance your well-being and empower you to take charge of your health.

Thank you for choosing *Ancient Natural Remedies Improved with Modern Medicine*. I hope this book has provided you with useful knowledge and inspiration to integrate ancient remedies with modern approaches to health. Your opinion is very important! I invite you to leave an honest review of this publication. Your words will not only help other readers discover this book, but also enable me to constantly improve. Thank you for your time and support!'

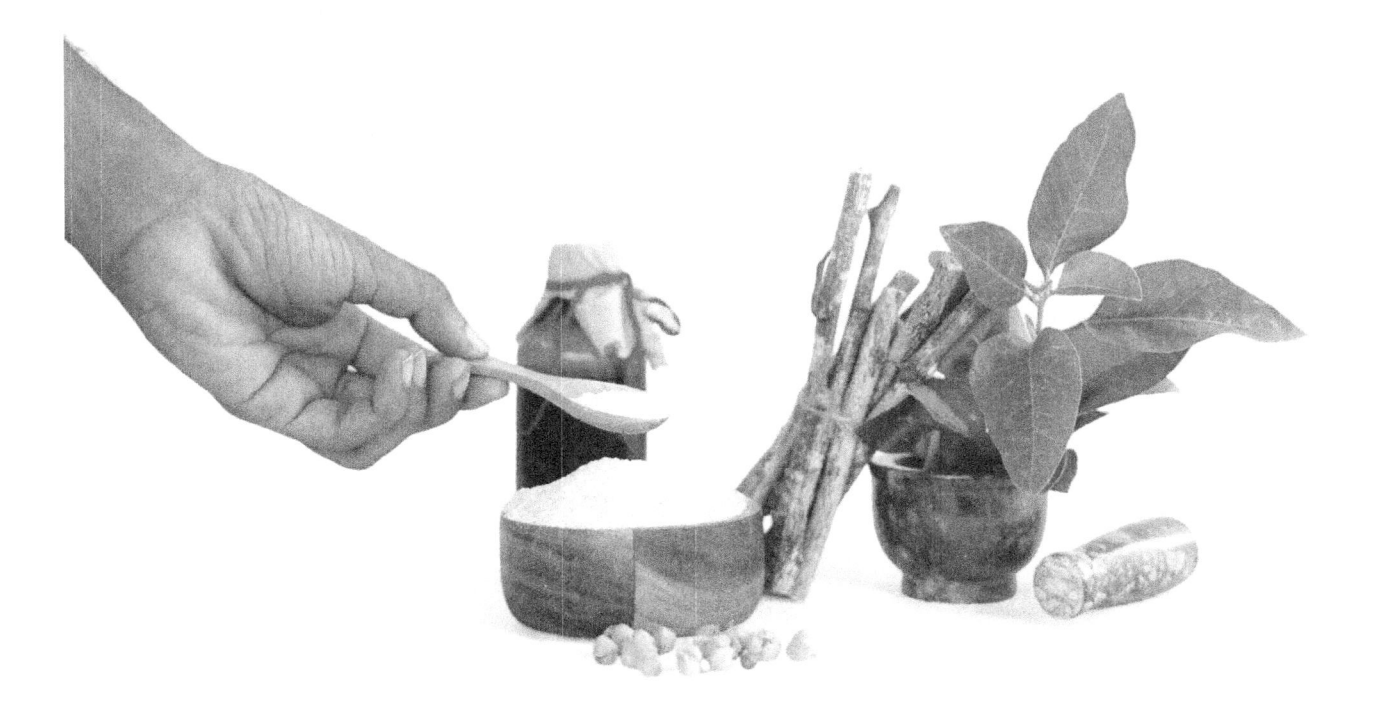

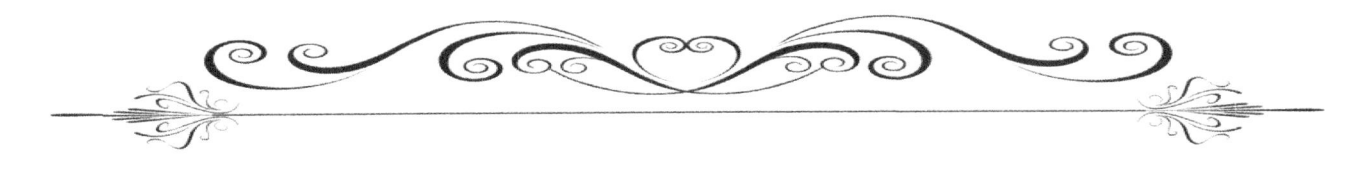

Made in the USA
Las Vegas, NV
28 March 2025